The Gift of Touch

By

Jay North

One Globe Press
P. O. Box 1211
Ojai, CA 93024
www.OneGlobePress.com

Writers Guild of America registration number #

VDMA1C92BAB7—2006

ISBN-13: 978-1463557607

ISBN-10: 1463557604

Fourth edition **revised** 2013

Printed in the United States of America

The Gift Of Touch

Therapeutic touch for health, energy work and bodywork has been around for thousands of years. As Jay North—author, social activist, organic farmer, practitioner of healing arts—believes (*with opened memory) for *billions* of years people have been able to heal themselves.

The Gift of Touch is an exciting new work intended to aid those seeking relief, improvement, and change in their quest for a more pleasurable life and their own contribution to the evolution of humankind. *The Gift of Touch* is intended to motivate readers to initiate positive changes in diet and physical activity that can result in improved physical, mental, and emotional well-being, and an overall lighter experience.

Jay believes that healing practitioners throughout the world have a unique opportunity through contact with

4

fellow beings to assist in the orchestration of change so that a shift in consciousness may occur. Jay's premise is that simply through the art of systematically touching and handling the body's energies, lives dramatically improve.

The focus of this book is the manipulation of energy FLOWS. Energy is what creates and holds in place the material we collectively refer to as reality. When energy flows smoothly and evenly, the body operates at its optimum level. An embodied being operating at an optimum level equates to a calm, vital, productive, happy individual in harmony with self and other beings, including plants and animals.

But, energy in and around the body tends to lock up due to many factors such as injuries, trauma, drug and alcohol use, breaks, strains, and so on. Locked or blocked energy is what tends to foul things up in the body and mind. In this book, Jay North reveals how energy in and around the body can be freed up to flow and to be of optimum use and value.

This comprehensive book is filled with interesting facts as well as step-by-step instructions in a variety of healing techniques, covering everything from esoteric concepts such as karma cleansing to basics such as how to give a Swedish massage (the most widely used and accepted modality in massage therapy throughout the world today).

Jay explores the release of entities (some call them *ghosts*; others *entities*, *mechanisms*, *implants*, the *Devil*, etc.). Jay's vast experience in the healing arts confirms that no matter what we label them, there is the existence of energies that are not ours, and he explores this topic with insight and his ever-present humor.

The Gift of Touch also delves into the areas of nutrition, fasting, standing meditation, group healing sessions, romantic love, massage for babies, and Native American sweat lodges.

There is an entire chapter devoted to sexuality and sensual massage. Jay asserts that a healthy sex life is one of the most healing therapies for well-being and overall happiness. He states, "Sex is one of the highest degrees of the expression of love we will ever find. For thousands of years, nations, cultures, and individuals have designed all sorts of interesting techniques for expressing love and sexuality with one another. Sensual massage does more than just relieve tension...it is spirituality—the act itself. It is two people coupling in order to bring pleasure into this life experience for and with each other." *This chapter is specifically intended for couples, not practitioners and their clients.*

There are many books about healing on the market. What is NEW is that this is a book that increases the reader's ability to be in Oneness and to experience One-ness in their daily experience of life here on this plane. *The Gift of Touch* techniques aid in the quest for "Beingness" and Oneness by removing the blocks to Oneness. According to Jay, "Our basic path is to return to who we truly are, nothing and everything, aware that we are the creators, temporarily, mistakenly separated from the one that created what we are in order to experience who and why."

In the chapter entitled "Rites of Passage," Jay covers the topic of assisted dying with sensitivity and

6

perception, examining how a healing practitioner can ease the transition from this plane to the next.

As Jay succinctly sums up his book, "The purpose of this work is to free people from their minds and allow them the experience of the "unfoldment" of the soul and the opportunity to expand into a world of Love, Peace, and Joy—a world without the need for wars, without insanity, ignorance, and compulsion to control or destroy. A world where man/womankind can live freely without the negativity of judgments and projections; where the only standing order of the day is one of goodwill and that you have a truly wondrous day filled with prosperity and joy."

The reader will find esoteric subjects such as wormholes, Grids, Cellular Memory Processing and Crack The DNA Code. While these may seem unusual at first, readers will do well to understand and apply these techniques to healing and the ultimate goal, the unfoldment of the soul.

> *"The Gift of Touch is real and is powerful.*
> *The world needs this book."*
> Crystal Morning Star
> Healing Practitioner for over 40 years

*Open memory= ability to recall

A note from the author

I am not a doctor or a licensed medical practitioner... but I do have many opinions on health, food, life style choices, and natural healing methods.

I have worked in Spirit Healing and as a writer on healing and organics for over thirty-five years. I do not offer prescriptions or recommendations, although I do share information. I always have. And that is my intention here. The sharing of ideas is both our God-given and First Amendment right here in the good old U.S. of A.

My purpose is to share ideas, data, information, beliefs, and opinions that I hold to be true; and that can lead anyone to a healthy, enhanced experience here on Earth. I am aware, however, that no two ideas are alike. We may agree on some viewpoints and choose to disagree on others, and in this way we will come to live in harmony. I fully understand that you may choose to disagree with many of the ideas put forth in this book; and while I encourage debate, I choose not to participate in debate this time.

Finally, please remember I wrote The Gift of Touch in order to provide information. In all cases where severe health challenges are an issue I highly recommend you visit your doctor or professional health care provider so they can help you make sound decisions.

I wish you good health, long life, and prosperity. Love, Peace, and Joy in your house, Jay.

Added Note to my readers:
The Gift of Touch is "Channeled" material, which is to say has come to me from sources outside of myself. While I do take full responsibility for the creation of this manuscript, the form in which it came is not always

acceptable to some readers. I apologize for any inconvenience in advance. I have left the words in tact as conveyed and this does not necessarily represent good grammar and choice of words in the proper English language. You will also see the use of humor and slang; and again I hope this is not a bother to my readers and that you will take this work seriously and apply it in your own lives as well as that of your clients (where practitioners are concerned). The words of "You," "Them" "One," and "We" Refer to various flows of energy we are dealing with. These practices, as you will read, can be applied to a client, to one's self, and to groups of individuals. This will become clear as you proceed through the materials.

My prayer is that you will come to realize the final outcome and help spread the joy of *The Gift of Touch*. Jay North aka J. Mountain Chief

About the Author Jay North

Jay's first introduction to massage and healing work occurred in beauty school. While studying cosmetology in 1968 he took a basic course in massage. This class primarily covered scalp, facial, hand, and foot massage but it was just the beginning of Jay's interest in massage therapy and healing techniques. In 1970, Jay studied at the Santa Monica School of Massage where he received his certification as a massage therapist. He next completed advanced training with Greta Schmidt from Germany, whose specialty is sports injury therapeutic massage. In the ensuing years he added reflexology, Do`-In, and Shiatsu; and became proficient in Reiki, Levels One and Two. Jay is a Certified Access Facilitator, Certified Spiritual Counselor, and a Certified Practitioner in Science of Mind. In 1990--1999 Jay studied herbal medicine under the tutelage of a shaman of the Blackfeet Indian Tribe, Leonard J. Mountain Chief, who also introduced him to the teachings of White Buffalo Speaks; a disembodied elder of the Tribe.

Jay's interest in the healing arts has spanned over 35 years in which he has read over 1,500 books on topics such as philosophy, psychology, specialty studies of the mind, spirituality, touch for health, the study of herbs in healing, life direction planning, nutrition, energy work and other related fields. *The Gift of Touch* has been a work in progress since 1976, with new, very relevant discoveries from 1996 to 2012.

Jay is also an organic gardener. He owned and operated *Paradise Farms* in Carpenteria CA for over twenty years, during the 70's through the 90's. Jay has a deep respect for the planet and assisting Mother Earth to heal herself.

Jay now lives in Ojai, CA. In the Chumash Indian language it means "The Nest."

Please share your experiences with Jay. Feel free to write Jay anytime. He really does answer his own letters. Contact Jay North through either of his website www.OneGlobePress.com

Help clear and save planet Earth. Please send your friends to any of the websites listed above and ask them to purchase their own copy of The Gift of Touch, Open Spaces, and Miracles in the Kitchen.

Thank you in advance.

FOREWORD

The Gift of Touch will aid those seeking relief, improvement, and change in their quest for a more pleasurable life leading towards the unfoldment of the soul and the over-all evolution of humankind.

Some individuals may have physical or emotional needs that require the services of medical professionals. This book on massage therapy and energy manipulation (healing with energy) does not replace the role of counseling or the occasional requirement of drug therapy or medical attention. This book is intended to motivate readers to initiate positive changes in diet and physical activity that can result in improved physical, mental, and emotional well-being— and an overall healthier, happier experience here on planet Earth and beyond. Look for your personal unfoldment to occur!

My hope and prayer for seekers of truth is that you will find this work useful and that it will be of value in your search for a healthy, happy, and complete life; and lead you to the ultimate outcome—unfoldment of the soul.

My prayer for you is the gift of touch—that all with whom you come in contact may receive from you the true gift of Love, Peace, and Joy.

Healing practitioners throughout the world have a unique opportunity to connect with fellow beings to assist in the orchestration of change so that a shift in consciousness may occur.

I would like to express my humble gratitude to my allies in teaching for the great and wonderful guidance I have received from each. Thank you, Christ, Vivekananda, Vishnu, Buddha, Hubbard, Mother Mary, Pammy, Sam, Leonard, Gary Douglas, Hazarat Inyat Kahn, Thich Nhat Hahn, White Buffalo Speaks,

12

and all the multi-talented in-bodied healers, practitioners and body workers I have come to know.

This book is for those seeking relief, change, and improvement in their lives and in Earth's conditions; and to those who wish to contribute to creating miracles in people's lives. Healing practitioners throughout the world have a unique opportunity through contact with fellow beings to assist in the orchestration of change so that a shift in consciousness may occur.

The Gift of Touch is a rewrite of my earlier work, *Advanced Breakthroughs in Massage Therapy* (1976). While the truth of energy and flows has not changed, I have had the opportunity to experience additional, relevant attributes. You will find them in this manuscript and they present a new perspective in providing the gift of touch to people's lives. This new perspective in providing touch can very possibly change and even save (cure) lives providing that we are willing to accept/allow change, improvement, and an enlightened awareness of one's body and field of conscious awareness.

Please visit Jay's websites www.OneGlobePress.com and www.GoingOrganic.com

Please make use of the American Standard Dictionary whenever a word appears that you do not fully understand.

Table of Contents

Introduction: Taking the Mystery out of "Alternative"

Over the past five decades, reports of new – and, in some cases, extraordinary – healing techniques have been widely publicized. This has had a very interesting effect on many people and on how they choose to take their medicine.

In the United States alone, there have been countless studies and research papers written on alternative medicine, health, and healing. Topics covered extensively in the past include acupuncture, Ayurvedic medicine, energy healing, vitamin and herbal supplements, meditation, yoga and deep breathing

As an exercise: Restrain from using any form of sugar for one week and replace it with fresh organic fruits, vegetables, grain and nuts.

exercises. But is all of this "for real?" Or, is it just "mind over matter?" Please stay with me; it goes much deeper than that.

Over four decades ago, the discipline of mind control – pioneered by Religious Science founder Dr. Ernest Holmes – and specifically Silva Mind Control, was developed to help relieve the suffering that came with illness and to help people come to a 'prosperity state of mind,' and even get rich if they had a mind to do so. And those techniques have persisted. They are more popular today than they were back in the 'good old days' of black-and-white TV.

Why are so many people looking for answers in

15

directions that go beyond the good advice of the simple family doctor when it comes to treating their disorders? Because clinical studies prove that miraculous healings do, in fact, take place without the aid of modern science or simply by "popping pills." People are waking up and looking into the cause of illness and disease, and taking responsibility for their own cures.

Let us examine just a few of the off-the-beaten-track healing modalities that are available to the people of Planet Earth today.

In Truth, "alternative" healing has been a staple of many societies since the beginning of time.

There is increasing evidence that in many cases, today's mainstream medicine is embracing the practice of alternative healing methods – whether they come from religious men, shamans, or therapists – by combining them with "traditional" treatments. For example, participants in the Benson Cardiac Wellness Program for coronary artery disease encounter relaxation response techniques that include prayer, meditation, and cognitive therapy. These patients have reported fewer symptoms of chest pain, less shortness of breath, less fatigue, fewer symptoms of depression, anxiety, and anger; lower levels of cholesterol and blood pressure, greater weight loss, and an increase in exercise tolerance; not to mention a feeling of overall well-being and a more active sex life.

So is there something here? Something we should be taking a closer look at? *Yes, there is*...and that is exactly what we are going to do throughout this book.

> *As an exercise: Try juicing fresh organic vegetables three or four times a day, drink eight to ten glasses of water, and see if you notice any improvement in your energy level, after just ten days.*

Are cures possible?

World-famous doctors such as Deepak Chopra, Andrew Weil and nutritionist Gary Null believe that such "alternative" cures are possible. They report absolutely amazing results employing healing techniques in use for hundreds of years abroad but go relatively unnoticed in the USA – or more recently have been suppressed by the American pharmaceutical companies. At the same time another set of ideas are just beginning to have an impact on the forefront of our society: that many so-called "necessary" surgeries and use of dangerous chemicals may not be such a great idea for the human body after all.

These doctors, along with countless thousands of others throughout the world, agree on this one simple, powerful principle: *"What we ingest affects our health."*

Are pills the answer?

What does the word 'antibiotic' *mean* anyway? It means *anti-life*. In this new millennium people all over the world have started to look into new *pro-life* approaches instead – approaches based on what's actually good for the body and can cure the problem in a way that sustains life rather than kills it. People are looking for ways to live not only longer, but happier, healthier lives with more vitality. They are looking for ways to sustain their bodies without the use of modern medicine or just "popping pills" as a means of restoring

17

good health after many years of poor diet.

Why? Because many of us are suspicious of pills and pharmaceuticals – and we should be. Just what *are* we ingesting?   Might those things be the *cause* of our problems, rather than the cure?   Could the things we take into our body – including the things that are allegedly good for us – be the reasons so many people are running to the doctor's office?

We will cover that question – and many others – very thoroughly throughout this book.

Aren't you just talking about "faith healing?"

Maybe I am, but maybe not.   Maybe it goes much deeper than that. A great writer named Napoleon Hill once wrote, "*What the mind conceives and believes; it can achieve.*" This is true to a much larger degree than many people believe, but it is not simply a matter of faith. It's a matter of physics.

Stay with me now, please.

Our Homo Sapien minds and our physical bodies are essentially made of matter, energy, space, and time…and the controlling factor, the factor that dictates our overall well-being, is **energy**.

Why is that? Because, *energy* runs the whole machine. Without it we have nothing. The planets, our bodies, everything, requires energy. Without it, the other three would not exist. It's as simple as that.

That's just good old-fashioned high school science. So what's the news? It's this: Correctly applied techniques for manipulating or controlling energy can allow bodies to heal, to regain their wholeness, and to live far longer than anyone heretofore thought possible. In fact, strictly through controlling energy flows, *we can live forever.*

We really *can* "achieve what we believe."

Way back in the late 1950's, L. Ron Hubbard said it as well. *"When you have a spiritual being that realizes who he or she is,"* he wrote, *"when that being realizes who's in charge and comes to recognize energy flows and his or her ability to run or control the energy of the body, then the body can go on living for a very, very long time."* And this can happen *without* the aid of conventional medicine, which Hubbard himself strongly opposed for most of his life. No intended endorsement of Dianetics or Scientology here, but the point is clear: You and I can indeed live very long, very productive, and joyful lives without the use of drugs that supposedly sustain life. It is, in fact, very possible that we can live happily for a very long time strictly by controlling various energies. This book is devoted to controlling your energy and that of your clients, to help improve overall health and longevity.

Juicing turns people around, 180 degrees

People like Gary Null, Jack La Lanne, Dr. Norman Walker, and many others have promoted the idea of extending life – and a very healthy life, at that – strictly by using fresh organic vegetable juicing, combined with good clean water and plenty of regular exercise.

People around the globe have been applying these techniques to their daily lives and living far past what conventional doctors have referred to as "terminal case life expectancy" – or, to put it simply, *dying at a predictable age.*

These "juicing" techniques address the chemical energy in your body – its acidity level as opposed to its alkalinity. The principles of a high green vegetable juice diet are based on the idea that fresh **organic** vegetables and fruit juices, good clean water, and deep breathing and exercise can change one's life; and may be all that one requires to sustain stamina and vitality for decades.

It has gone well beyond theory and into practice ... and this practice apparently works well for millions of healthy people running around today.

Shamans from many cultures have applied what we are just now learning

Our ancestors knew about spiritual healing centuries ago. They lived in connection with their spiritual

> *Caution: Avoid mixing too many modalities at one time. Make a selection, choose the route to wholeness that FEELS right, and stick with it for a period of time. There is always opportunity to change.*

essence and used natural herbal remedies in the treatment of severe challenges to the human body. A study of the ancestral wisdom of Native American culture reveals that spontaneous healing has occurred in what some consider a 'suspect' manner.

Science, and our faster pace of life, has ruptured our relationship with nature but it is possible to reestablish that harmony and be healed completely of some very troubling diseases strictly by reconnecting with nature. As an old shaman I once knew, named Leonard J. Mountain Chief, a Blackfeet elder said, *"Healing is available to anyone. All one has to do is to get out of one's own way and let the nature do the work."*

There are many routes to wholeness

The list of alternative supplements, herbs, homeopathic remedies, vitamins, and healing modalities are endless, and the choices are many. What is required, especially in cases of severe challenges, is *research* and *evaluation* so you can make the correct decisions based on personal beliefs, hopes, and dreams...and by determining what is really going to work for *you* to sustain your optimum health.

Already the little voice in your head is saying, *"But, he/she is my doctor. If alternative medicine is so great why doesn't he/she prescribe it?"*

Good question! Many contemporary doctors don't know about the many choices available in the world today, and some may not care to know. But others *do* know about the many roads to good health and well-being that a patient can travel today, *in conjunction with* western medical modalities for treatment of disease or discomfort.

Listen to what the "traditional" doctors and practitioners say ... but remember it is your **personal responsibility** to seek out what you *FEEL* is the best route for your body, your health, your life, and your longevity.

21

Here is a short list of alternative methods available for your consideration:

- Energy manipulation or energy healing

- Therapeutic Massage

- Acupuncture

- Chiropractic Treatments

- Herbal remedies

- Fasting and diet changes

- Organic fruit and vegetable juicing

- Meditation

- Sweats and water purification

- Drumming and soul retrieval

- Vitamin supplements

- Deep breathing exercises and relaxation

- Prayer work or positive affirmations

- Touch for health

- Hiring a personal fitness trainer

- Counseling to resolve past issues

- Past-life regression therapy

- Movement through dance

- Gifting through touch

…and the list continues to grow.

This book focuses on energy and how to manipulate it to help create over-all change and improvement in the aspirant's[1] life.

The choices are many. What works? It *all* works. The only choice that is important is the one *you* make. Only *you* can decide if alternative medicine really works! That decision is *yours*.

At the end of each chapter, I have included a list of questions students have asked me while discussing the material presented in that chapter. The student questions are in italic font with my response shown directly below each question.

---

[1]   Aspirant = one who chooses to seek the unfoldment of their soul

Chapter 1 – The Art and Science of Healing

To the practitioners of healing arts and sciences, it is no secret that massage —touch for health, energy manipulation and bodywork on several levels — has been around for thousands of years and, in truth — with Opened Memory[2] — for billions of years.

Many cultures and civilizations have understood the value of being-to-being body contact. The focus of this treatment is the manipulation of energy FLOWS, which we cover thoroughly in, Part Two and Part Three of this book. Handling and dealing with energy flows and blocks allows one to experience shifts which create relief and overall improvement in one's life and vitality.

Energy in and around the Body — it's All Energy

What is energy healing?

Many people today are at least aware of the terms Chi, Pronic Healing, Reike, and Healing Touch or Touch for Health. Through the media, and through acceptance of relatively new healing modalities, people are learning about the benefits to applied energy manipulation. One day, it may even become a household term. In Power Touch therapy, we go after (in order to facilitate healing) very specific areas and some considered

---

[2]   Open Memory = Ability to use recall at free will for your entire life tract

rather esoteric. We practitioners consider these esoteric areas vitally important to address.

Healing with the manipulation of energy flow requires a practitioner to handle or deal with one of four components of the Physical Universe. When we become involved with handling issues that block wholeness and well-being of body, mind, and spirit we are working with matter, energy, space, and time.

While counseling, psychiatry, and psychology work with matter (significances), energy healing works with flows, locks, blocks, and barriers. The whole idea or concept is to remove various blocks and assist one (a client) to come into a new, rehabilitated, or re-naturalized, state of being.

In energy healing work, we consider the primary factor for healing to be "energy." Energy healing moves energy, and, in that consideration, we are able to bring about healings. In doing so, people's lives are forever changed.

As an example, we work to resolve problems or challenges; work to restore optimum health; work to remove communication barriers; and so on up through a wide range of issues for people. We work to find a way to lead one to a higher form of life, living a pleasurable joyous life with restored abilities. Energy healing is simple in form and practice, easy for anyone to learn and provide loving service.

As for energy, one may wonder, "What exactly is this invisible stuff?" Energy is what creates and holds in place the material we collectively refer to as reality. While it is true that our perceptions — thoughts, opinions, beliefs, considerations, decisions,

25

conclusions, projections, judgments, and so on — add solidity[3] to our condition, it is the change of energy in those perceptions that can bring relief and improvement and decrease solidity, allowing one new found freedom.

Specifically, we are talking about energy in relatively scientific terms. Energy does few, but very definite, things: It flows; it gets blocked or locked; or it disperses (moves in general and non-directed ways). We can free energy that is blocked or locked in and around the body so it can flow and be of optimum use and value to the aspirant. So, we have energy that flows easily and effortlessly. We also have the conditions of locked or blocked energy, dispersed uncontrolled energy, and energy that flows in tune to individual's optimum health and vitality. Energy in and around the body can tend to get locked or blocked due to many factors such as injuries, trauma, drug and alcohol use, breaks, strains, and so on. Locked or blocked energy is what tends to foul things up in the body, mind, and spirit. When energy flows smoothly and evenly, the human body operates at its optimum[4] level. An in-bodied being operating at the optimum level equates into a calm, vital, productive, happy individual that is in harmony with self and other beings, including plants and animals. Likewise, as we strive to harmonize with others, we can also have unwanted energies and the energies of others. I will discuss the energies of others in a later chapter.

Various interesting things can occur when the body

---

[3]   Solidity = mass/weight, to be solid

[4]   Optimum level = level which is best, of most value, and of highest productivity and joy

receives treatment to bring about change. The individual can go through a series of gradual changes that may not be very dramatic or even very noticeable. On the other hand, in some cases, there may be rather sudden shifts that can be somewhat surprising and unsettling to even the most advanced practitioner and aspirant. Individuals may experience unexpected emotional highs and lows, body twitches, or sudden aches and pains. Some feel an immediate sense of relief — an improvement that seems miraculous without having gone through the expected hardship of an arduous climb towards the seemingly impossible. Some feel forever changed and emerge with a sense of Love, Peace, and Joy for life; and a renewed sense of compassion, purpose, peace, and responsibility.

Energy from being to being can be pushed, pulled, flowed, drawn, forced, implied, begged for, stolen, and even bought and paid for. Energy can be shared. Energy can be exchanged, as in exchanging money for goods and services. Money[5] is energy, is it not? Energy can be manipulated and unwanted conditions changed for the better with the proper handling of energy flows.

Simply through the art of systematically touching and handling the body's energies, lives can be dramatically improved and people can finally come to a place of the highest understanding.

An important ingredient is the practitioner's attitude and direction of his or her personal energy flows — a subject I will cover thoroughly in the next chapter.

---

[5]   Money = a tool used for exchange. It is nothing more than energy we use to exchange for more energy

Frequently Asked Questions and Answers

What do you mean by manipulation of energy flows? I mean, energy is invisible isn't it? How can someone handle and manipulate it?

While it may be true that energy is invisible to some, others do see energy, as in being able to see auras and such. Many healing practitioners can see the energy of dark spots, light areas, blocks, locks, and barriers.

For the second part of your question: Can energy be manipulated? Yes, most definitely it can be. We, as spiritual beings, can grab hold of energy and channel it. Please be patient with me and I will get to this in more detail.

Can you explain this in "baby terms" please? This sounds great, but I'm not sure what you mean. You make it sound like energy has substance, sort of like matter.

Energy is not like matter at all. It is only one part of the four units that make up what we collectively refer to as Matter. Matter has mass and significances; energy has charge and wavelength. Energy can be turned on, shut off, dispersed, locked and contained in a vessel for a period of time, and can be manipulated to bring about a desired result — as in clearing an individual from problems, upsets, and so on.

Chapter 2 – The Practitioner

Compassion, Love, Peace, and Joy are the finer attributes of healers, practitioners, body workers, and light workers. What appears to be "real life" (which tends to be illusion) hands us a variety of different qualities as we journey through life. We manage to run into all kinds of emotions and attitudes: hate, fear, jealousy, pride, envy, greed, hostility, and all sorts of unwanted sensations and emotions coming at us at a rate that at times is somewhat uncomfortable and at other times nearly intolerable. Yet, it's all part of this complex game we created. Yes, many naturally evolved people experience Love, Peace, and Joy in abundance with ease. Many seem to be gliding through life with little or no baggage at all. These people used to be rare but many are now starting to take responsibility for their spiritual evolution. We have come to find there are ways out of mental energy traps and a way to the unfoldment of our souls. This comes about through the manipulation of energy flows, deep breathing, meditation, prayer work, and an individual's focused concentration.

Your responsibility as a practitioner (during a session) is to create and outflow energies of the highest quality — Love, Peace, and Joy coupled with Compassion. This is not for the sake of protocol but for the desire to bring forth the outcome you want for the person you are working with.

Years ago, when I was in the cosmetology business, I worked in a salon in Beverly Hills with over 30 employees. There were several personalities to work with: temperamental hairdressers, manicurists, shampoo people, assistants, receptionists, and, of course, a demanding clientele. One of the most valuable lessons the owner taught me at a very young age was that no matter what you have going on in your life — bills, relationship problems, hopes, dreams, and fears — put them all aside when you walk through the door. Put a smile on your face and pretend you absolutely love everyone.

Good advice, and not far from the truth in looking upon the appropriate mindset of a healing-arts person. This is <u>important stuff</u>. With enough out-flowing of positive energy you can change your client's world — and yours at the same time. The energy that you process outwardly during a session — and in life for that matter — is the energy that contributes to creating this very interesting game here on planet Earth. The energy and words we use to create what is, is what creates what is. Gossiping and talking negatively behind a client's back or that of a friend even worse creates disharmony and a less desirable experience — and helps lock us further into the traps we have created. That's why "everything equals everything, created by what we think, say, agree on, and vibrate into our planet Earth reality. By our words, acts, and energy we create what IS, and we will get to that much deeper later in this book. Stay with me now, it gets easier and more fun as we go along. Create and outflow the experience you want for your client and they will receive it. The same holds true for your own life and you will learn simple processes to deal with your own energy as we go along. Yes, to a certain degree you are responsible for your client and their condition. Take the time and responsibility to meditate on and outflow the experience of Love, Peace, and Joy. Your clients will love you for it and they will continue the flow out into the world; thereby bringing about change to the planet and everyone on it.

It amounts to unification of thoughts, feelings, mind, and heart coming together for the purpose of flowing loving energy. This is easily accomplished with quiet meditation or visualization, and simple processing. Do this: Recognize your higher, essential self and blend with heart, mind, and body.

Try this simple exercise: Point a rectangle away from your body at a point three feet from your body. Visualize the creation of Love, Peace and Joy, coupled with Compassion, and outflow this creation to your client. Direct this energy flow towards their third eye and towards the heart Chakra. Gently allow the flow to enter into the realm of your client's heart and soul. This is soul healing at a very high level and effective form; and it may be all you need to do for a session to be complete. If your client appears complete then end the session at that point! How do you know if the client is complete on a subject or an item? By the way the client looks and feels and by what he or she has to say. Have a good look at the client's Aura for color and clarity.

Love, Peace and Joy will heal this planet.

Frequently Asked Questions and Answers

Do you mean that I, or someone else, can make good things happen just by thinking good thoughts about them?

Yes. You can help guide a person into a good or better space and assist in their healing with your attitude and out flow.

31

What do you mean by 'the third eye'? I'm honestly not trying to be funny, but it must be something we can't see so how do we know where it is so we can direct energy to flow to it?

The third eye is located directly on your forehead between your eye sockets.

I looked up the word Chakra and the dictionary said "Wheel". I don't understand what you mean by the heart having a wheel. Would you please explain?

Sure. It is a wheel or an axis if you will. Chakras are energy focal points on the body. From the top of your head (being the crown Chakra), move downward and you will locate the third eye chakra, throat chakra, heart chakra, solar-plexus chakra, and root chakra. There are others in your hands, feet, knees, lower back occipital area, and shoulders, back of the knees, ankles, fingers, and toes. All total there are 22 chakras that can be located on the body and used to create harmony or disharmony.

Chapter 3 – Where Energy Gets Locked in the Body

Energy can be locked anywhere in the body. The most common places are the extremities. Therefore, the hands, feet, and head are the areas to check first. Why is this? It appears that these areas are points of implants[6] of our own design (which means purposely created). Areas also worth checking are the spine, the scalp, facial muscles, solar plexus, and all internal organs. The body may be trying to rid itself of unwanted conditions by pushing blocked energy away from the body.

Energy blocks can occur as a result of injury, trauma, or drama. Injuries occur in a wide variety of ways. For example, virtually anyone or anything — a car, horse, motorcycle, paintbrush, baseball, or mop — can cause an injury. An injury can leave an impression on the body for a very long time (lifetimes, for that matter). And, of particular importance, Energy Memories (or Energetic Memories) can be stored on a cellular level[7] for many lifetimes, until the being —or a practitioner — finds a way to eliminate the unwanted blocks or unwanted conditions, usually through processing.

Blocks, locks, barriers, and items you pull off the being

---

[6] Implants = forced considerations, conclusions, beliefs and postulates. Either agreed to or resisted upon, they are what entrap a being into not knowing

[7] Cellular memory and cellular memory processing will be completely covered in chapter, Cellular Memory Processing pg. 123

feel heavy. You, the practitioner, will feel a particular vibration, heat, tingle or heaviness in the palms of your hands. When items you **pull** cool down, (cool down means the item has no charge left on it) you will not feel these sensations any longer because they will have dissipated. The charge[8] is then gone completely; which means the item will not have an effect on the client's life any longer, or, at least until the client re-creates "IT"; a subject we will cover completely later in the book.

The memories that lie deepest and contain a lot of power are those of emotional drama/trauma. These are lies, betrayal, invalidation, forced emotion, and withheld love and affection, just to name a few. On a more esoteric level[9], there are also implanted items that should be dealt with — and deal with them we shall.

These blocks have a grip on our lives. How we think, speak, and operate is directed by how we are feeling and by our ability to cope with and to rid ourselves of unwanted conditions; namely energy blocks, implants, and energy conditions of other origins. The practitioner will find that many blocks contain fear, anger, grief, death, and dying.

While this writer understands and appreciates the efforts of any good doctor, when being treated by a

[8]   Charge = an item that contains negative energy blocks, locks, and barriers. It also refers to the amount of attention given or drawn to an item by the client. People with fixed attention tend to have a lot of "charge" on a subject

[9]   Esoteric level = the deep or high levels of processing that lead one to the final goal — practiced in many cultures as mysticism.

physician it just may be worth one's time to explore alternative methods to healing, as in massage therapy and energy manipulations. And, it just might be worth the good doctor's time to investigate NEW ways to bring patients closer to good health — Love, Peace, Joy, and HEALING in a quicker, less expensive manner that is also less supportive of the pharmaceutical companies and less invasive. For that matter, some Holistic practitioners may choose to work on a donation basis (this may not be right for all).

Relieving energy blocks, i.e., held-in considerations, stuck conclusions, and a whole host of other illusions, is a simple matter of application and practice. In essence, energy blocks are simply illusions ingrained into a client's psyche so strongly and inherently that the client cannot rid him/herself of them without aid from you, the practitioner. What makes these concepts illusions? Is it that they are a lie and we have the choice to simply rise above them? Until we reach that ability, we must process ourselves through the maze of insanities that could have an adverse effect on our lives.

What I am offering here is a route; a method; for releasing pain, discomfort, and suffering from all sentient beings — allowing their experience and our own to be easier and more pleasurable. This method is not the only way — perhaps not always even the best way. Things change, and I don't want to be one who says facilitators *this is the only way*. The work should be a thing of Joy, relieving hardship, aiding in the possibility of total abundance, Peace, Love, and Joy for life and the lives all sentient beings.

Through forgiveness of our sins we shall discover everlasting peace and joy. Through the healing of

35

misbalanced energy we shall live in perfect Love and harmony. The only sin is to allow the continuation of the MIND[10] to think it is in control.

Frequently Asked Questions and Answers

Can this sort of thing be done without the person's knowledge or permission?

Yes, it can, not for harm, but for good. Let's say you are walking down the street and you notice someone in pain or hungry. If you happened to believe in a God outside of yourself, wouldn't you say a prayer for that person? It is really the same principle here, only you are reaching out with a flow of Love, Peace, and Joy and emanating that set of ideas towards the person you are hoping to assist. Quite simple, isn't it?

Now, on the other hand, if a person you notice is walking a path or on a journey and having a difficult time figuring out their life or path I would not invade their space but allow them to figure out their own outcome. I would never cheat a being from experiencing exactly what they need to on their walk through life.

This sounds like an invasion of privacy in some ways and yet a good one if being done for the right reasons. What concerns me is can someone misuse this also?

---

[10]   Mind in control on a cellular level; individual organization; unit; generating charge on cellular memory level; the Mind has no real control. True control lays hidden deep within the being him/herself.

36

There is no misuse. We are here to do good works and make a contribution. The only intention here is loving service.

If someone or something in him or her is fighting against this sort of thing, what determines who wins?

As long as there is improvement, if there is gain, if there is release from suffering, we all win — as One.

Chapter 4 – Unlocking and Channeling Energies

Manipulation of energy is a simple process. FEELINGS direct it more than thought. It **does** require one to open and expand his or her intuition and physic abilities.

With eyes open or closed, visualize the flowing of energy. Some can effortlessly accomplish this by seeing light fields, hot or cold spots, and dark masses. We may detect blockages, auras, injuries, disease, misalignments, and so on. What is necessary for you and your clients alike is NOT to attach too much importance to anything one finds and, regardless of the mass or appearance of power, to continue working and get the thing you're after. Even if an apparent evil entity rears its ugly head look at it as a good thing. You're about to handle a huge block for, or with, your client. Staying with this process occasionally does require resolve and determination but, because of the ease and enjoyment of doing the work, you should not notice much difficulty in getting through the processes[11].

Always stay in communication with your client by asking questions and particularly watching for indications of change such as shifts, rises, and falls, lightening, or solidity. Start with a very simple explanation of the process and try not to go into long dissertations of how or why. Allow for questions and answers but keep this brief as well. Following a short introduction, bring the space to a calm and safe place using your intention. Ask your client if he or she is comfortable and if they

---

[11] Process = a period of time devoted to handing negative life energies

require any change or improvements in the space to help feel more comfortable. Ask the client if music is desired, lots of light, or low, dim lights. Since you are going to be giving a massage, your client will need to disrobe or not during an energy (clothes on) session. Remaining partly clothed is acceptable during massage, and all the appropriate parts may remain covered with a sheet or towel. Leave the room while the client removes his/her clothing (when giving a full body massage only) When you return, knock gently on the door before entering to be sure the client is ready.

I always recommend light music during a session. Again, ask if this is acceptable with your client. I prefer soft lighting and no interruptions of ringing telephones, and I do not answer the door once a session is started.

Do not assume anything! Ask your client why he or she is there. You may see other things going on with their energy but this is of no importance. What is important is what the client is doing there in the first place. Ask your client, "What brought you here? What can I do for you? What changes would you like to have happen? Can you allow changes in your life?"

If a person does not require or desire a change then no amount of work you do will have any lasting effect. Yes, you will bring temporary relief and some relaxation, but for long-term or semi-permanent change to occur the being must want it. Not that temporary relief is bad — it beats no relief at all.

With eyes first opened and then closed, observe your client. Open up to your intuition and visualize what needs attention. Look at your client (actually see the person, body, and aura). Visualize having completed a job well done — see the result you want as being complete even before you start. Quietly, without seriousness and fanfare, do a silent meditation, bringing heaven and earth together — mind, body, soul, and call in higher spirit. Meditate on Love, Peace, and Joy, and, with the help of all GODS, deliver (flow) that energy to your client, directed towards the third eye and heart Chakras. Simply flow the energy. Do not attempt to push, force, or feel a need to tell anything. Just flow Love, Peace, and Joy.

Touch the body. The Gift of Touch is real and powerful. Use it well. Remember this, my friends: Enlightenment includes, by definition, the word *lighten*. So lighten up. Have a good time. Tell a few jokes. My very best advice to my beloved friends is dance; sing, and laugh — laugh a lot. Be Merry or be Joe. It doesn't matter. What *does* matter is that you and I become less 'matter' and more FUN.

Beginning Gift of Touch in Massage Therapy

To begin the initial process just walk around the person's body lying on the table (that's the client lying on the table not you — I don't know why people always ask me that, but I just thought I would clarify it before you called to ask). Now, lay your hands on the body, firmly and confidently. Start at the feet, work the legs, and keep moving up until you reach the head. Don't leave out the arms and hands. Pay extra attention to toes and fingers. Ask the client to turn over so you may work both sides of the body. This is simply to get the communication going, to put yourself in communication with your client's body and your client in touch with his or her body and the fact that someone is touching it.

Keep verbal communication going, but not to the point that it is distracting or irritating to your client. Ask, "How is it going? Is this pressure OK? Is there anything you would like to talk about or tell me?" This is an important feature of the session and requires your devotion, attention, and ability to listen without interruption or the need to do the talking. Allow the client to do the out-flowing and just keep listening and referring to what he/she has to say. The more you allow your client to talk, the more they will tell you, and this is an essential aspect in allowing you to handle the energy of what comes up through their telling. It is sort of like a confessional, except you are dealing with the energy of the words, not the words' meanings or the mass of what is apparently being projected, except to relieve mass (charge, polarity) through the process of energy manipulation.

Get a flow going. Again, energy in and around the body does various things that can have an overall effect on a being: It flows nicely; it gets locked up; it disperses in an uncontrolled fashion (i.e. hyperactivity); and it can be sent elsewhere. Moving and manipulating energies is what this work is all about — to get a flow going that is most beneficial to your client's mental, physical, and spiritual well-being and enhanced life experience here on Planet Earth. I feel the best way to get the most desirable flow going is with the application of massage and, as will be later discussed, through simple turning of polarities.

When this part of the session feels complete you will then know you have gotten in communication with your client, his/her body, and its requirements. You are ready to go onto the next step.

During this next part of the practice, the client should be laying comfortably on his/her back with a round pillow under the neck and a bed pillow under the knees. Continue to ask, "How's it going? What's happening? Anything you would like to say?" But avoid getting into a conversation. This isn't visiting; it is a treatment session with the intention of improving and changing the life conditions of your client.

Again, start at the feet. Apply firm pressure but not to the point of pain or causing discomfort. No Pain, No Gain is B.S., at least in this context. Another thing you need to watch for is how many traumas the body has experienced and how much mental torture and abuse the being has endured.

Always start with the extremities — the head, hands, and feet, as this is where a large amount of blocked energy is located. This is where you are going to get a lot of release — feet, hands, head, neck, scalp, fingers, and toes. Take your time. Spend the time to do the work completely in order to release as much locked energy as you can. You are *not* going to get it all in one session. Forget the notion of changing a person's life completely and forever with just one session. It won't happen and you will only disappoint yourself if you expect it. This is not to say that miracles do not happen, they do, but just be patient in all cases.

Work the feet completely for a fair amount of time or until you notice a shift. A change may be subtle and it is your job to recognize it when it occurs. Noticeable changes are fluttering eyes, twitches, changes in skin tone and color, changes in breathing, coughing, outbursts of laughter or crying, and a change in the client's willingness to communicate. Note the appearance of relaxation and rest the person is getting during the session.

Continue to work the extremities: hands, feet, spine, head and neck. The work you do with the head, face, and neck can be some of the most significant so pay particular attention to what is going on in these areas. The head apparently also contains a lot of mass, i.e. points that hold a fair amount of charged energy blocks. You can press lightly on the head and scalp, or you can give a deep massage. Remember how good it feels to go to the hairdresser and have a really nice shampoo — that's how the head massage should feel to your client. Work the entire head, neck, scalp, and facial muscles, paying attention to the third eye and occipital areas. What those two areas have in common for a lot of people is that they tend to hold a lot of power in the form of considerations, opinions, ideas, conclusions, judgments, agreements, projections, and so on. This is the stuff you're after; this is the work itself, clearing away **stuff** that we have been carrying around for a long, long time. Stay in communication[12] with the person you are working with because there's a good chance that when this stuff starts to fly off your client is going to have a lot to say.

How long do you need to spend on the extremities? It varies case-by-case. It might take a half an hour to cover the areas described above or it might take three hours. We (groups of light workers and healers) are finding however, that this stuff dissipates quickly. This is why it is important to keep your client talking and to observe what's going on.

It is a conscious action to send released energy off to

---

[12]   communication = the exchange of ideas between two points, and with attention and intention, equals understanding

another dimension. Simply tell it to go and send it where you might. In truth, it does not take much effort. It *does* require intention and a decision on the part of both the practitioner and the client to let it go and send off unwanted energy blocks, locks, and mechanisms that neither the client nor the practitioner desires.

Where does this energy go? It goes wherever you send it. Send it to another dimension. Send it to a lockbox in the desert. Send it to a benevolent source who won't mind handling it. Some send unwanted blocks to GOD — as in, Let Go and Let GOD. Send this garbage to a higher intelligence and allow it to be gone, without the need to re-create it. Whatever it is, just let IT go. That's advice for you and your client!

To continue the release processes begin working the inner abdominal area. Use a good old Chinese standby: Work the tummy deeply in circular motions. Go as deep as client's level of comfort and acceptability will allow. Use clockwise and counter-clockwise motion from the ribcage down to just above the pubic area. This is very therapeutic work as well as instrumental in releasing many energy blocks. You are clearing a lot of physical mass; thereby allowing for easy passage of materials that need cleansing from the body.

Once you and your client have achieved a sense of completion and you have released your client's locked up stuff you are now ready to handle this dispersed energy. This jumble of rattled, loose, uncontrolled megahertz, dispersed stuff may remain with the body and could tend to stick elsewhere. *(Student question: Can't the practitioner do something to prevent this? Reply: Yes, sweep away unwanted or undesirable energies; send them off to another dimension and allow them to be gone.)* This is energy that you can calm and make to be flowing. In this way you are creating a flow to the betterment and overall improvement of the client's health and well-being.

This is a two-way operation. You are pulling junk off *and* putting back lovely intention. You and your client are in-flowing and out-flowing energy simultaneously. When there has been enough energy exchange for one session and your client displays improvement, end the session.

Frequently Asked Questions and Answers

What do you mean by evil entities? Are you talking demonic possession or something like that?

Yes, something like that. There may be a presence that has intentions that are not to our benefit, such as destroyer's entities. There are two points here: First, try not to agree with the entities, and secondly, do not resist them. By your agreement or resistance, you are giving them power. We will cover this in a later chapter.

If the client has come to you for treatment, yet something in the client seems to be fighting against what you are doing, how do you know what the client really wants?

Go after what is for the client's own good; find it, and deal with it.

If you determine that the client really doesn't want the healing, yet you feel that it would be for their ultimate good and that they will be glad later, how do you determine what you should do?

Never work with someone that does not resonate with the healing or does not want the work performed with them. Never work with an intoxicated person. The only way a person gives up drugs or excessive drinking or makes changes in their lives is because they choose to do so.

Chapter 5 – Swedish Style Massage

Swedish style massage is, by far, the most widely used and accepted modality in massage therapy throughout the world today. The reason I feel it is so effective for this work is that it easily creates the flow we're seeking.

Swedish massage involves gentle touch and manipulation of body tissues and the reorganization of energy flows throughout the body. It is one of the most easily understood and easily applied massage techniques available to massage therapists and healers of a wide variety of modalities.

For some practitioners it is a simple question of intuition and a feeling for the work while others require formal training to get the basic essential movements to giving a really wonderful Swedish massage.

It is highly recommended that all massage therapists take the time themselves to have this work performed. It is essential to get a real FEELING of what feels good and what doesn't.

The practitioner should use a light, rhythmic touch and be consistent. Apply massage oil or cream for added ease of working the body tissues. One can use a wide variety of manipulations to facilitate the results one is seeking. There is kneading, as in kneading dough; there are appropriate stretches; pushing and pulling of the muscles; or turning and mild stretches of the head and neck while very light pushing and pulling on the spine and working of the rib cage.

Work from toes to head on both sides of the body.

Remember, you are working to free and change energy conditions in and around the person's body, thus allowing for an enhanced experience of your client here on Planet Earth, a place not so easy for some to experience — more on this in later chapters.

Once again, starting at the feet, work up the body towards the head. Work slowly and rhythmically using even pressure, and without changing pressure or rhythm too often. This requires skill and practice except for those practitioners who have a keen sense of how to handle the body and an instinctive sense of what good touch feels like.

The massage process may take an hour or more. You will be working on both sides of the body, back and front. You may wish to indicate to your client to take several deep breaths during the massage, or, at a minimum, to pay some attention to his or her breathing. Keep the communication going. Ask frequently, "How is it going? Or, what's happening?" Also ask, "How is the pressure? Too deep? Not deep enough? Would you like me to change the music?" Staying in communication is the point. Remember, it will be easier to read your client by listening, and there will be nothing to hear, if you don't first ask!

The massage is important in relation to the energy work you are doing, and, in fact, you are carrying through with the energy manipulation treatment by giving the massage. (We will get very much deeper into this subject in the following chapters, just stay with me for now and it will become very clear shortly.) Now, you're simply evening out the energy flows and releasing more stuff as it comes up. While your client is laying face down on the table pay particular attention to the spine.

The spine is another one of the sticky areas where masses and other things tend to get locked. There are different spots for every person. Some experience lower back problems while others have problems in the mid-back or neck.

Gently, yet firmly, move these energy blocks away from the spine. Place your fingers next to the spine, pushing inward, down, and away from the spine all at the same time. This easily accomplishes the task of removing blocks locked on the spine. You're sure to find a lot of locked energy on the spinal cord — take your time and get as much as possible but remember; it just isn't going to happen all at once. You're going to be seeing this person more than a few times so take your time. Swedish massage can take years off one's age. Do more than a so-so job and your client will forever love you. Speaking of which, of course, you have been flowing Love, Peace, and Joy to your client during the process!

Another place on the body to pay close attention to is the face and facial muscles. Why? Because, they too tend to hold a lot of locked up charge. Using these same gentle techniques, work the entire face. Work all the muscles and pressure points on the face, hairline, scalp, ears and base of the neck deeply and smoothly.

You will be amazed at how much heavy stuff you're going to rid your client by working to remove long-left masses. Masses are, in fact, cellular junk piles more felt than seen; although some practitioners recognize them very easily. Be sure and work these areas well.

Note: You may want to try this visualization: Ask your client to visualize a two-way energy flow moving through their body from head to toe, up and down and

49

out, smoothly and slowly, ever so softly. The energy can appear in any color desirable to the client, or as clear light. The Energy flow can help move off undesirable energies and locks, or the energies of others—a subject we're about to cover.

Frequently Asked Questions and Answers

Does a massage therapist have to have a special license and training to do this sort of thing? Can someone just study from a book, declare him or herself a massage therapist, and hang out their shingle so to speak?

Yes and Yes. Most massage therapists have special licensing, although in some locations one can be a massage therapist without a license. I think we have way too many protective laws in this country as it is. Certainly, you will want to check with your own state of residence to be certain.

Couldn't someone damage someone by pushing on the wrong places?

Yes, but this is highly unlikely to happen. The client will let the therapist know for sure!

Chapter 6 – Introduction to Turning Polarities

"Who the hell is this? I just don't feel like myself these days!"

If the above two lines sound familiar, it is because we all experience stuff that just doesn't quite feel right or just doesn't feel like ourselves, right? We all have had the experience of, "That doesn't sound like me and it doesn't feel like something I would say or do". NO? It isn't.

This subject gets into an area that some, particularly fundamentalist religious types, do not want to talk about or even know about. It gets into spirits and the spirit world. If you don't want to know about these topics just skip this chapter and go on to the next. I won't be offended.

Some call them *ghosts*; others call them *entities*, *mechanisms*, *implants*, the *devil* and about a hundred other not so endearing terms. No matter what we label them, there is the existence of energies that are not ours. There's a good chance that when we feel a little off it is not our own energies we are experiencing. As a matter of fact, 75 percent of the time we are getting hits that do not belong to US! (Student *Question: What do you mean 'getting hits'? Reply: Bombarded by energies that do not belong to us!*) It could be age-old stuff we have carried around for a long time; or it could be a recently acquired energy that just happened to be floating around and it resonated and stuck. The wide range of the type of energies that can attempt to have an impact on our lives is endless. They range in volume and strength as well as personality influence. Whether ghosts, entities, implants, conclusions, contracts, projections, opinions, goals, sadness, joy, money, work, being-ness[13], creativity, peace, hates, loves and a whole host of other deluded decisions; what they are or are not is not nearly as important as the fact that we don't need them or any influence that causes anything else to be other than who we truly are.

Being-ness is one of our main objectives (more on this later). This subject is nothing more than energies and is nothing to fear. Energy is energy and it is all moveable. We have the ability to change our lives and to be responsible for our actions.

We can pull other being-ness and pivot the energy. Then we can draw back the native energy for optimum use.

The responsibility you take for this work can certainly help any being be exactly who they are and increase their personal responsibility, control, and happiness in their lives. Please, just try not to get too hung up in all this other energy stuff. It is not very important and is easily handled by releasing, pushing, pulling, and, in general, manipulating energies to a desirable FLOW. The procedures described in earlier chapters are the procedures used to clear energy not belonging to the client. It is also easy to apply off-body work, the subject of the next chapter.

Pull off ghosts, entities, and other being-ness and intentions by sweeping your hands over the client's

[13]   *Beingness = the causative creation of be, the willingness to be*

body (or yours for that matter), and simply sweep them away. This will become a very simple process for the practitioner who learns to manipulate energies well.

Frequently Asked Questions and Answers

You mean you think there really are ghosts or whatever that come in to people's bodies and inhabit them? Sort of like science fiction beings from another world?

Yes I do.

Could this be what is going on when the doctors' say someone has multiple personalities?

Yes, most definitely.

Do these ghosts or whatever always mean harm to the person? That is, do they want to take over the person's body and be "top dog"?

No, not at all. Many of us have disembodied beings hanging around us to help guide us through this maze. We need to shake their hands and talk with them more often. If Christ or the Buddha appeared to you today, would you turn your back on him or would you invite him in for a cup of tea?

Chapter 7 – In and Around, Up and Down — It's All Energy

This chapter covers handling energy by expanding the sphere of interest. We simply widen our interest and work on stuff in and around the body by pushing and pulling. In fact, we will be handling many issues with/for our clients with off- bodywork. In part two of this book, you will be handling entirely energies with off-body work (see Chapters 20-26, pgs. 70-102).

What does this stuff feel like? It feels different to different people. Many feel heat, slight tingling, or a vibration, all of which may be very subtle or quite intense. Try this: Rub your hands together firmly and quickly for a minute or so, and then stop. Now hold your hands about an inch apart and FEEL the heat, tingle, or vibration. This is the sensation or feeling you will get when performing the following processes. If you do not feel much at first, don't worry too much about it. Open up your intuition, close your eyes, and do it again. Practice a couple of times and you will soon get it. There is nothing mysterious about this and nothing wrong with you if you don't get it right away. You will be able to feel this stuff on others and clear it. The vibe that you feel after the rubbing test is the feeling you are going to feel while pulling and pushing energies with/for your client. At times it may feel quite intense. Other times you may feel just a very slight amount of charge. That is because there may not be much charge on a subject, or the charge is cooling off. When a subject goes cold, it's done. Leave it alone. On the other hand, if it's hot then stay with it - whatever it is - until it cools down. Again, try not to get hung up on what it is and do not attach more importance to the thing other than just to get it cooled off and gone.

How do you know it's gone? By the way it *FEELS*. The procedure for working off-body is, in truth, quite simple and easy for anyone to apply. The work does not require psychic ability or the power to see the extraordinary. The work is done by simply sweeping with your hands off and inches away from the client's body. You can sweep until you spot a dark spot or some sort of charge that feels like it does not belong. Once you find a subject, no matter how icky it feels, just stay with it and it will cool off and have less charge and less impact. One can remove a lot of stuff that needs to come off just by sweeping the body.

Continue to run your hands over the body from the feet to the head and the entire aura, and expand out as far as necessary. When you have handled a fair amount of charge; the client appears complete; and the client communicates a change for the better; it is definitely time to end. Be sure to schedule a follow-up session to handle anything missed as well as new stuff surfacing and ready to come off.

Note: If you notice that I use the words Need and Want often, and you feel that is not 'OK' because of a popular new age concept that Needing and Wanting are somehow unacceptable, this is exactly what I mean about attaching too much importance to words, subjects, and phrases. Try not to attach too much "have-to's" to this subject. It will take the fun out of it!

What about doing these processes from a distance?

Yes, this work can be done from any distance. Many of the people I work with today are not in my home state and I can work/pull off anything from anywhere. All you, the HEALER, must do is find a connection to the person you are working with. Hold your hand or hands out; pull energy from the being until you find the connection, then start to pull off specifics. Ask for higher self or guidance to find the exact thing to extract. End these sessions by blowing the charge out of your environment and asking the client to set a new decision in the Here and Now to guide their life to a fuller expression of who they truly are—more on this in latter chapters.

Frequently Asked Questions and Answers

What is an aura? I've heard of it, but I'm not quite sure.

It is an energy field around the body. It has been photographed many times.

Can you make a mistake and "pull off" and send away something that really belongs in or around the body?

No and yes. That which belongs will feel good and will not come up as something that needs to be turned and gotten rid of. The client, or you for that matter, will not release that which is pleasurable. A "ghost" may be sent off; and if it turns out that it was Casper, well, then, that's a whole other story.

Who is really in control, you or the client?

The Client always is. You are there as healer/facilitator.

Chapter 8 – Standing Group Healing Meditation

Simply relax and pull what needs to come off

Re-alignment, re-construction, and re-activation can be applied by anyone who aligns to and tunes him or herself in to the vital power with this work. For practitioners, I recommend keeping explanations of this procedure short and to the point. There is never a requirement to be the talker—instead, be the doer. The treatment speaks well for itself and if your client doesn't get it then a lot of talk won't help. This treatment hates a lot of jabber. Approach it with reverence and silence—it's golden. Following the session please do allow for the experience to be shared. Encourage a brief discussion between you and your client of what occurred. Some will not want to speak. Others won't be able to.

I have seen many stories and people who have experienced rather dramatic changes after these sessions. I have seen cancers come off, Aids relieved, heart problems cease, depressions disappear, money problems solved, relationships repaired, newfound good luck and good fortune revitalized, and a whole huge wide range of major changes and new personal discoveries made by those who have participated in Standing Meditation healing sessions.

Standing meditation, group healing session

Lights low, healing music softly playing. A small group

of clients stand in an informal circle. Instruct your clients just to allow their body to move (if they like) gently with the music. The process is done silently. There is no verbal communication. Instruct the clients to relax and allow the body to move in whatever way it wants.

Breathe and relax—always start by asking clients to breathe and relax

The practitioner or practitioners move quietly throughout the space to make contact with each client individually. With eyes open or closed, hands approximately three to four inches away from the client's body, and with open palms, practitioners should move their hands slowly around the entire body of each client. Allow yourself to *feel* the energy blocks and situations with each client concerning their bodies and difficulties. Pull off whatever needs to come off (become a vacuum) and pull[14] off whatever you find, sending this stuff to another dimension. Open your crown Chakra and blow off whatever comes up and off and OUT. When things appear to be calming down or lightening up, assist the client's body to realign itself. Check for diseases, dark spots, entities, mechanisms, implants, projections, judgments, and other apparent malfunctions. Whisk them all away. Clear the body and the aura. Send whatever you find to another dimension, or to a lock-box in the desert.

To complete this session you need to clear the air. Clean the space; sending all undesirable energy to another dimension so as not to allow anything removed

---

[14]   pull = to remove

to stick to another entity (client).

Work to re-align, re-structure, re-create, and re-activate the client's energy, body structure, and operation to the highest optimum level. The entire process could take several hours to complete, depending on how many bodies are in the space and how much stuff the practitioners find to remove. Encourage all participants to stay until all are complete. Clients may want to have Swedish massage soon after this procedure. Again, be sure to clean the space before departing. I'm not taking about physical trash, I am talking about mass[15], but you knew that, didn't you?

The practitioner's only outflow during one of these sessions is Love, Peace, and Joy.

May we leave the place better than we found it.

Frequently Asked Questions and Answers

You spoke about entities. Is it possible for an entity that you have pulled out of someone to get out of your control and enter someone else?

Yes, this can happen. If an entity finds another body in which it resonates it will attempt to stick around. Just pull it and ask that it find its own home.

Is there some special thing that you do before you start these group sessions to protect yourself and all clients from any possible evil entities that might be around and

[15]   Mass = heavy energy containing weight, form, color, taste and smell.

might emerge?

Yes, thank you for asking. We can speak the following words:

Dear Mother Father God,

Come to us in this place,

Bring us into our highest good,

Shower your loving protection over us,

Dear Heavenly Mother Father Shower us with your loving presence,

Bring us to a place where we come to know you,

And in this place, we ask to be blessed with your loving light and guidance and healing,

Deliver us your power for the highest good,

So that we deliver your Love, healing, and goodness.

And now we begin.

Chapter 9 – A Change of Pace: Interior Cleansing

And you certainly may need one after all this — a change of pace, that is!

There are many types of treatments for benefiting ourselves. One worthy of consideration is interior cleansing.

We have the opportunity to consume many harmful substances, both intentionally (drugs, alcohol, food activities, fast foods), and unintentionally (pesticides, herbicides, fungicides, chemical fertilizers, gas fumes); not to mention (but I will, of course) those little pesties that manage to make it into our foods and eventually into our stomachs: WORMS! Oh, no, not that! Oh, yes. There may be over two hundred and fifty classes of pests occupying our bodies at any given time. There are, in fact, religious cultures that actually believe that ridding the body of worms rids oneself of the devil (the Master Serpent) itself.

The practitioner's responsibility in assisting a client to rid him or herself of parasites is guidance. To be an effective practitioner to others you must first be an effective practitioner to yourself.

At times, we all may have a little trouble sticking to a regime—and this one isn't easy even for the devotee of fasting. This regime requires ingesting supplements to kill off parasites and restoring one's internal balance. While I cannot recommend or prescribe any supplements I have heard through the grape vine that wormwood, black walnut, burdock root, mugwort, willow bark, black cohosh, and yellow dock are perfect for cleansing, as well as chaparral, pau d` arco, and oil of oregano.

Doing a cleanse releases unwanted entities

There are several completely safe and organic methods for fasting and the elimination of parasites. I would advise that one find a very competent health professional to recommend safe products for purchase at a reasonable price from almost any health food store. While you're at it, if you have a medical doctor, it is worth a checkup just to make sure it is advisable for you to go on a rather specialized cleansing.

In any case, if you decide to do a cleansing be sure to drink plenty of clean, high-quality water and use plenty of living acidophilus following the treatment.

An interesting little thing that may occur with some folks is sudden mental and physical changes. We can easily handle some of these by ingesting the right herbs and vitamins to aid in the realignment of functions we take for granted or which require a little attention from time to time. A good idea is to recommend to your client to have a relaxing massage during a heavy cleansing, not only for relaxation but also for help to keep things moving, if you get my drift.

Be sure to include a change in diet during a regime of cleansing. You may wish to consume plenty of dark green and red **juiced** organic vegetables. Grains, seeds, and nuts are also good to include at this time. It might also be advisable to quit meat, milk, cheese, wheat, citrus, white sugar, eggs, and, of course, all drugs, alcohol, and smoking while cleansing.

Also, some people might want to consider doing some sort of cleansing or fast once or twice a year based on personal requirements of health and enhancement. Good indications a fast or cleansing may be in order are: yellowish skin tone or eye color; poor skin condition; nail and hair quality and strength; heavy tongue with lots of build up; continuous bad breath; persistent gas in the tummy; heavy appearance in posture or facial expression; chronic depression; aching back or bones; chronic colds or flu; lots of fatty tissue on the skin; etc.

You and your client will just <u>know</u> it's time to clean house.

I give you the fruits of the forest so that you might enjoy them

I give you water that it quenches your thrust

Eat the fishes of the sea

Delight in the fowl that take to the air

Consume the beast if you must

Have a good fast; it will help you

To see me more clearly.

<u>Frequently Asked Questions and Answers</u>

What do you mean by clean, high-quality water? I'm

right on the town water system so I know it's clean, and I always let it run for a few seconds so that it isn't something that has just been sitting in the pipes.

No, I'm sorry, but your tap water is not clean water. Drink distilled water. There are many high quality water-purification systems on the market today.

I thought worms were something people in foreign countries who were malnourished got. You make it sound like anyone could get them.

Yes, it's true. We all get worms. They come from organic produce, fish, and pets. We can even pick up parasites from people through intimate contact.

Chapter 10 – What Does Sex Have to Do with Healing?

If the subject of sex bothers you in anyway—don't read this chapter.

I don't really need to ask that question, now do I? Whoever doesn't believe sex is healing, please raise your hands! Sex and sensuality. How many books are there on the subject? So why do I find it necessary to bring it up here? Because I love sex—and so should you. I don't mean to sound presumptuous but let's face it folks, a healthy appetite for sex can be one of the most healing things you can do for your life, well-being, and overall happiness—as well as that of your mate's.

Again, this may look like a departure from healing but just hang on for a moment, please. This is for couples, not for practitioners and clients. Nevertheless, it is an important ingredient.

We're not talking about sex without love merely for the sake of the sexual experience. No, sex is one of the highest degrees of the expression of love we will ever find. For thousands of years nations, cultures, and individuals have designed all sorts of interesting techniques, (i.e., the Kama Sutra and Tanta), for expressing love and sexuality with one another.

Start by flowing to your partner LOVE, PEACE, JOY, and add Safety, Warmth, Compassion—the pure ecstasy you get being with your partner.

Loving massage for the enhancement of sexual experience

Lights low, music on, light wine chilled, room designed with love in mind, clothes on or off. Don't forget the anticipation of unwrapping the package to find morsel treats!

Sensual massage is creativity. It is joyfulness. Hell, its fun! Each partner must do his or her part to make this a wonderful experience for the other. Don't leave out feathers, oils, and all other interesting enhancements you can dream up on your own!

Sensual massage is very light touch. It's OK to touch. Please do it more often, even if it doesn't always lead to lovemaking. Touch your mate with love and kindness, and by all means make it SEXY. I hate this part—as though I would even have to mention it, —but please, don't go right for the genitalia. Why rush it? That only displays immaturity. Take your time to do a lot of nice kissing. You're not going anywhere, right? Use a nice, light fingertip touch. Run your fingers all over your partner's body. Use your tongue a little or a lot. Use flowers, use a feather, riding crop, a carrot, whatever you and your partner deem appropriate. LOOK: this is your space, your life, and you and your partner's sexual experience. Why not enjoy it to the max?

Sensual massage does more than just relieve tension as some of my contemporaries believe. Sure, it is great for relieving life's stresses—to a much higher degree than just the orgasm function that occurs as a result of pounding two bodies together. Yes, it is spirituality— the act itself. It is two people coupling in order to bring pleasure into this life experience and to aid in the realization of who they truly are. Wonderful, loving beings ought love to display closeness, as in Oneness. Some entities just can't stand this much love. So? Do it more often! Make them really mad! Anyone who tells you that "sex is dirty," "don't do that or you'll go blind," or any other misguided, misinformed, mistaught lies — please, just ignore them.

Sex and sensual massage are beautiful and in no way can be done incorrectly. The best teacher is your partner. Listen well to what he or she has to say and have the courage to do what he/she wants. Although he or she will most likely reciprocate, this isn't about *what's in it for me*! It's about what we can do to further our "We"-ness and is a totally pleasurable experience that we can have here and now right on good old planet Earth. For more tricks of great loving sensual massage, visit a really cool adult store

Gypsy Star, from where you are the moon shines upon you

With great delight I take flight in the plight of not having you

In my arms tonight we will not fight nor struggle

For in this moonlight that you have brought so bright

You have removed all fright

Now in your sight

We can delight in this loving union

And with all our might make love all night

Gypsy star, you are the stars sun and moon.

Chapter 11 – Return to Oneness

The concept of Oneness is nothing new. What may be NEW is your ability to be in Oneness and to experience Oneness in your daily life. *The Gift of Touch* techniques described in this short volume of work should aid in your quest for beingness and Oneness by removing the blocks to Oneness. That is our basic path; to return to who we truly are, nothing and everything; aware that we are creators temporarily separated from the One that created what we are in order to experience who and why.

Krishnamurti referred to this thing as *cosmic consciousness*. The great Hermities called it the *all in all*. Hubbard referred to it as *source*. St. Michael to *I AM*. Christ said, *"We are one in GOD,"* and Buddha taught us to find the *middle way* and our *essential self*.

Remove all blocks to Oneness simply by sweeping them away. Repeat, "I am One, we are One."

The path may seem hard

The mountains high

But with each step we take

The climb back to the one becomes easier along the way

You are my father

You are my mother, you are my sister and you are my brother

My teacher, my friend, and never my foe

You are the light that shows me the way

You are the LOVE that gives me life and the food that feeds my soul

We Are One

You are my father that gives me hope

You are my lover that strokes my hair

Without you, there is no life

You bring me to this place to get know myself

Knowing you does this for me

You are my sister who protects me along the way

My brother, you have brought so many GIFTS

Thank you for the love you give to me and the love you allow me to share

We Are One.

The wonderful Master Thich Nhat Hanh

Teaches us to notice our breath

Breathe in; my body is the living body of the living Christ

Breathe out; my body is the living body of the living Buddha

Breathe in; my body is the living body of the living Christ

Breathe out; my body is the living body of the living Buddha.

We are one, we are one, and we are one.

ALA hue ahla la hue ahla ahla.

And from my brothers and sisters, the Blackfeet natives from my beloved Montana

Ah uh hop vista doogy

Vista doogy ah hee

God Bless you God bless us all

I am One,

Frequently Asked Questions and Answers

What do you mean by Oneness? Are you talking about being complete in myself or do you mean some sort of Oneness, combining with all that exists to reach some sort of total Oneness or completeness with everything else that exists?

We are all One, separate entities connected through spirit.

71

Chapter 12 – Healing One's Self

The power to heal one's self

Dear Mother Father God, give me the power to change the things that I can and the intelligence to accept the things that I cannot change.

It is as though some sort of built-in mechanism gives us the right and the willingness to suffer if we so choose, but remember the word <u>choice</u>!

It has been postulated by many popular philosophers that allowance/acceptance, or rather the ability to simply experience whatever it is that we are experiencing at the time (which can include suffering, joy or nirvana) will aid us in our quest for Happiness and Joy. Yes, simply through allowance[16] we can, and just might, meet up with God.

The ability to stand firm and allow all emotions—anger, fear, pain, jealousy, joy, etc.—to be without the need to change anything can help bring about the changes we desire more quickly than if we had struggled to create those changes. It is all about the choices we make, right?

Many great teachers have concluded that everything is perfect all of the time, even though this may sound outrageous, especially at times of extreme difficulty and pain. The function of acceptance is to teach the students of this life the experience to grow in insight

16   Allowance = allow to flow, allow to occur, willing to experience

and awaken to the essential self, also described as the Great I AM: GOD/GODDESS within.

We homosapiens have the opportunity to experience, allow, accept, and, most importantly, to love exactly who, where, what, and how we are at the exact moment of NOW. And we can truly love the experience with the mindfulness of perfection and thanksgiving.

Love the experience and move on.

Imagine, if you will, a situation, any situation. Doesn't matter what it is, so just make one up. Create a moment of discomfort. Get a really good, solid mental picture of the thing with FEELINGS such as weight, mass, color, form, smell, taste, emotions (including pain), discomfort, unpleasant thoughts, decisions, and so on. Allow whatever comes up to come up. TRY not to stop a perfect opportunity for experience and expansion.

Example: Here I lie in my bed tonight full of fear, anxiety, and worry. The pit of my stomach aches. My body feels heavy. It's hot. My mind wanders aimlessly. I feel fearful, lost, and upset. GOOD. This is a great place to start.

Allow the higher source of all life, your guides, Christ, and all benevolent powers, to join you in your quest to experience this pain completely.

Lie face up. Take a few deep breaths, and rub your tummy in both directions— clockwise and counterclockwise.

Focus from your third eye or your heart. Allow yourself to experience this thing entirely with all sensations and emotions—and now flow Love, Peace and Joy directly into the center of the thing itself that you do not want— the pain, the sorrow, the hurt you are experiencing and wish would just go away. Love it, accept it, and allow whatever is there to exist without the need to make it go away.

Now, just continue flowing love and thanksgiving for the opportunity to experience and grow. Continue your deep breathing and gentle touching of your body; allow whatever comes up to come. Put in your courage and your willingness to allow this process to complete.

A shift may happen ever so subtly, or you may experience huge relief, or, again, just a very mild shift of energy. Also, the pain or whatever can feel worse. It may turn on a bit and that's OK, too. This is compassion. This is love. This is joy in the highest. When a shift occurs that appears to have lightened things up, (and it will, trust me!) end the self-application treatment. Acknowledge yourself for a job well done. You can do this treatment daily.

A shift will occur; I guarantee it. The experience of acceptance/allowance happens and feels comfortable. You're clearing stuff that may not be wanted. Then what, you ask?

This may not be a quick fix or it may be miraculous; and since we're all perfect beings there is nothing to fix anyway. NO, it's an opportunity to experience exactly who and what we are in the now and to allow shifts to occur in order to facilitate our expansion on this plane, which includes optimum health, vital well-being, happiness, and longevity. Remember, we only get sick and die because we believe that is the intent or the MIND has tricked us into believing in that reality.

Allow change, <u>without the need to re-create the thing again</u>. Remember, the mind is a wonderful thing to waste. The noisy little bastard may automatically try to re-create the stuff you would rather not have. This is an experience of choices. Experience the choices you want. Decide on what it is you really, really want. Picture it, feel it, and vibrate it[17] as though it were here now and allow that. Boy, what a change! Can't seem to do that? Fake it till you make it. *Smile and the world will smile with you.* In other words, keep practicing; keep trying.

This is a rather simple process. Whenever you are feeling icky, or have a situation or thoughts you would rather not have, such as illness, pain, or mental drama, simply go into allowance and acceptance and experience it completely. Flow Love, Peace, and Joy to whatever it is. TRY not to make this an arduous process. Keep it free of effort; for the harder you try, the harder it is to experience the desired changes.

Dear GOD, thank you for allowing me this experience.
Thank you for the gift of life and all it has to bring.
Thank you for my body. Thank you for the Source to all life that I may experience and grow to be all that I am.

Frequently Asked Questions and Answers

What do you mean, we only get sick and die because we want to, or are tricked into expecting to? Are you saying that people only die because they think they're supposed to or something?

[17] Vibrate it = create the energy vibration by the way you want it to FEEL

Yes! We become ill based on our thoughts, projections, and ideas about good health and well-being; and/or resistance to getting sick; or as self-punishment and debasement. We are not victims. We get what we get because that is what we believe we were supposed to get. Resonate with it, vibrate it, and bingo there you have it – well-being or disease!

I thought we were supposed to reject the bad things that come to mind. You make it sound as if we're supposed to embrace them and experience them and that's good or something.

What I am asking you to do is to allow the feeling of whatever it is you are experiencing and allow it to pass through, not to accept it. Nor should one resist that which they *FEEL* they do not want. By magnetizing it with resistance it will grow. Breathe and allow the unwanted to dissipate.

Chapter 13 – The Words We Use; Pivot and Release

A great Philosopher (Paramahansa *Yogananda)* once said that words have power. There is truth to that statement, and clients and practitioners alike will profit by becoming conscious of the words we use.

Combine energy with the words used and we have power whether written or spoken. We can box ourselves in or set ourselves free by the words we use. How? By repeating words and phrases we increase or decrease our freedom and ability. You know the negative words: *can't, won't, could have, would have, and try, not smart enough, not rich enough,* the list goes on . . .

Many of us manage to get ourselves into all kinds of therapies, treatments, exercise programs, diets and other healing modalities and therapy sessions. We spend hours, months, years, and sometimes a lot of cash. And, occasionally, we notice that things don't seem to change much! Why is this? What can be holding the things in place that we would rather not have? WORDS! And the energy behind them.

I am not suggesting one go out and buy every book that was ever written on the subject of positive thinking or attend seminars on "thinking your way to riches" or on healing for that matter. But thinking—the energy of thoughts, words, and deeds—certainly does shape our world.

After clearing a lot of unwanteds (no such word? Yeah, check your dresser lately?) for your client or for yourself, readjustment of outflow will be in order. It is

am—please see my book, Spirit Filled Prayers and Affirmations.

Chapter 14 – On Fear and Resistance

You have what you have because you wanted it or because your fear of the thing was so great that it created itself—because there are no accidents, right! There are no accidents based on the fact that we vibrate into experience exactly what we get. Countless philosophers have recognized the power of fear and resistance and our power to create the very thing we fear through the mere attention we give to it or the *resistance* to the thing itself.

It appears to many people today that there is some sort of a disease of suffering; a commonality of circumstances that is somewhat less than appealing. And a whole lot of people are experiencing a similar set of circumstances at the same time. How does the manifestation of dislikes occur for so many at one time? Krishnamurti referred to it as cosmic consciousness. This could be a correct answer but is there a way to break the chain and release the whole cycle of being connected to things we don't want? Yes, there is hope!

What are these undesirable conditions? What do they look like and how can we free ourselves of their impact on our lives? The range of complications entering the new millennium appears to be money or its lack, lack of control, depression, sex and relationship issues, confusion and lack of purpose, and the question of will the planet survive? These, among others, seem to be the central areas of concern. They range in volume and impact. The weight, mass, and emotions vary but the amount of stuck attention is very similar for a lot of folks.

How can I make the claim that you wanted it? You proclaim, "I don't want to be miserable!" No? Then why are you?

From the multi-millionaire who suddenly goes broke to the mentally ill person in the streets walking around mumbling to themselves we all choose our experiences or resist them to the point of self-creation. Why we make the choice is an individual thing, but make the choice we do. Even to resist!

Resistance creates undesirable effects by energy magnetism. It is very much like South and North Pole attraction. More aptly put, when we resist we get what we *most* do not want!

There is one more factor playing a role in what we experience and that is the FUN we get out of creating a GAME for ourselves. Yes, a game: "How-much-pain-and-suffering-can-I-create-and-endure?" Many of us might find this game on planet Earth boring if we did not somehow make it more interesting by creating all kinds of havoc. Then we check for survivors and casualties, and race around and struggle to repair the damage. Nevertheless, it still has to do with creating a game and the choices we make and the experiences we invite, fear, and resist. I don't mean to come off as unsympathetic to people's needs, upsets, and problems but there just might be a way out; or a way to solve these dilemmas: Stop resisting what you don't want.

On the other hand, things are **not** all bleak. Many beings have succeeded in rising above what appears to be a negative cosmic consciousness. How is that? Freedom of choice! And still others find a way to manifest themselves right out of it. But many people require processing to help spot and relieve (turn polarity on) resistance to whatever they might be experiencing.

The practitioner's task is to recognize and reverse the negatives. These are the fear and resistance choices made by the client; and this is providing, of course, that the client *wants* to change the direction of these forces and make new choices to guide their lives into the future. It is essential that the client see choices as positive or negative for a change in polarity to occur.

The procedure for relieving fear and resistance-based problems is the same as karma cleansing a topic covered later... Get as much of this stuff (charge) free and moving from the extremities as possible and then sweep the body for blocks. Ask the client to examine the things they have feared and resisted. These are the things they did not want to attract or things they did not want to have happen in their lives. Don't worry about what comes up. Remember, this is about moving energy, relieving impact, and allowing change to occur in the client's life.

Continue sweeping the body. Check the head, neck, and abdomen, as these appear to be the areas that contain the bulk of this charge.

Special procedure for handling resistance energy

Ask your client to visualize holding in the palm of their hand their fear or resistance. Ask the client, "What do you now own that you once feared and resisted?" Have them look into their own palm and ask, "What does it look like? How much does it weigh? What color is it? What emotion is connected to it? Are you sure it is yours? Who does it belong to?" Ask the client to describe the thing as much as he/she can. Just keep pulling energy as the client does the talking. Sometimes a simple procedure of sending it off will suffice but in all cases you should turn polarity, release, and discount for/with the client whatever the subject was that they held in their palm. Turn polarity[18] on each item (thing) they brought up.

The charge on the subject will decrease or slip away completely. Ask the client to make a new choice in the Here and Now.

Sweep the body, the aura, and clear the room or space; sending this energy off elsewhere. This can be a dimension the client instructs or one of your own choosing. Ask the client if he or she can go on through life without the need to re-create this charge, situation, or dilemma, and it will not impinge on his/her life any longer.

Frequently Asked Questions and Answers

Why would anyone want to make a choice to suffer? That doesn't seem logical.

We are here to experience and know we can survive and prosper. Some of us simply want to experience as much as we can and we do not differentiate the experiences until we are in them.

_____

[18] turn polarity = all subject have polarities, i.e. good and bad, dark and light, and so on. Turning polarity causes charge from polarity to dissipate completely.

We are all making choices—all day, every day. Once we are conscious of the choices we make we will live lives that are closer to the optimum idea we have for our lives and that of our fellow beings. Choosing the life we want requires one to remove old, buried thoughts, ideas, and postulates and to set new direction in one's life.

Following resistance processing you can perform a really great short Swedish massage for/on your client—clothes on or off.

Wait a minute? No accidents? Are you saying I wanted a car to hit me? I thought the drunk driver had something to do with it!

We manage to resonate what we get by our vibrations. We may not have wanted it exactly but we vibrate what we get through either fear or agreement and/or resistance. We may not want to experience the pain we suffer but we do manage to vibrate it into our universe.

So if someone is sick it's because they choose to be? That doesn't make sense! I mean, why would someone want to choose to have cancer for example? Or even if they did, simply saying "I wish I had cancer" wouldn't make it happen would it?

1) Resistance! I hope, I pray, I don't get cancer.

2) The deeply built in agreement to suffer—a subject we will cover later.

3) Now, cancer is a whole other subject. Cancer is just a life form trying to find a body. It does not realize what it's doing by destroying the body it has occupied.

Cancers can also enter through bad diet, which is choice. Cancer can come to one while under a great deal of stress or through resistance to cancer, yet another choice.

So handling resistance energy and pretending to hold it in one's hand and picture it will get rid of it and everything will get better.

Yes, it can, and will. Try it sometime. You just might be shocked and surprised at the effectiveness.

You mean we can make our lives a utopia simply by pretending that they are?

Yes. Smile. "Fake it til you make it "and" the show must go on". Okay, enough clichés` already. Yes, imagine the life you want. Picture it, and write it out completely. Focus your attention on it and allow it to come into being the way you want it. And so it is . . .

Chapter 15 – The Purpose of this Work

The purpose of this work is service in the light of true service to all sentient beings everywhere and elsewhere.

We sentient beings require a reason, a purpose, for our very existence. In the highest order, purpose brings us as close to our natural state as we can come.

Note: Dear Reader, you may notice throughout this book that I refer often to "it has been said" or "some of the greatest thinkers have said"; this indicates that the data has come from a source other than myself. Please refer to the list of thanks at the beginning of this book.

People are harried, nervous, self-centered, non-caring, cruel, and hurtful. No, no, this can't be true! Can it? OK, people are loving, caring, and sharing—giving without thought of self for the higher purpose: "WHAT'S IN IT FOR ME?" People are benevolent creatures who rarely consider themselves first and are always looking out for the other guy. Yeah, RIGHT!

Somewhere in the middle is the truth. My hope for the practitioners, facilitators, healers, and therapists of this planet is to take this work and all modalities that facilitate changes in people's lives. Go out into the world; do good works; flow Love peace and joy to your family, friends, and all creatures. Work for the overall benefit and survival of the planet and give to yourself freely (and yes, of course, accept remuneration).

My old friend Bucky Fuller used to say, "There is enough to go around for everyone." He was referring specifically to money, and why not? IT'S TRUE. There is enough *energy* going around for everyone.

As a facilitator or a healer you and I have plenty of energy to go around. Give it freely. *Flow Love, Peace and Joy out into the world wherever you go.*

This is the work of the compassionate, the caring, and the giver—the changer of conditions on planet Earth.

I had a roommate once who was the perfect example of love, compassion, and giving—without ever; even once, embracing the thought *"what's in it for me*?" He gave his love freely to everyone he met. He knows how to spread Joy and what it means.

Pamela V. North is another perfect example of loving, giving, and sharing. She passed over to the Other Side in 1998 but she was another perfect example of the perfect listener. Always the perfect listener to many a hurt soul who just needed to tell it all. She would listen freely for hours on end and never said once, "Oh, it will come back to me!" No, she gave freely, naturally, 100 percent of the time. She truly helped change and enhance people's lives. And when it came time for her to leave her body hundreds of people came to say goodbye and thank you.

Acts of giving, loving, sharing, and compassion come freely to some while others have to learn it. YES, I know what you're thinking to yourself right now. *Does the man expect me to work for nothing?*

No, not entirely. Not all of the time would be my answer. Do your good works—give Love, Peace and Joy freely. Take donations from those who can afford you the favor of support in order to continue the work you do to facilitate people's quest for salvation. *And allow* prosperity into your life. Feel it (vibrate it) and it will come.

The purpose of this work is to free people from their minds and allow them the opportunity to expand into a world of Love, Peace, and Joy—a world without the need for wars; without insanity; ignorance; and compulsion to control others or destroy communities. A world where humankind can live freely without the negativity of judgments and projections; where the only standing order of the day is one of goodwill for a truly wondrous day filled with creativity, prosperity, and joy.

Remove blocks to purposes by sweeping your hands over the client's body. Call up blocks and locked, hidden purposes. Check the head, heart, feet, and hands. Pay close attention to the heart and solar plexus. Ask for times of failed or denied purposes. Continue pulling until all charge on this subject cools down and ask the client "what is your purpose in Life?" Give the client several weeks to come up with the answer (no, you are not continuing the process the whole time). Finding one's true purpose may not be an instantaneous result. It requires asking and patience.

Dear Practitioner/Healer: My prayer for you is that you *find purpose in all that you do and are.* It is my desire that this work will align with the purpose you have in this incarnation, and that your passion will shine. Remove all your own blocks to purpose and let your light shine.

May the spoken word of Love, Peace, and Joy go out into the world and the entire Universe to aid in all sentient beings' quest for healing and self-realization.

Frequently Asked Questions and Answers

Do you mean that we can actually help people just by listening to what they have to say? We don't have to try to come up with the answers to their problems in order to be of help?

We do not have answers for people with questions. Only they have the answers— of course, as does The Creator.

So just moving ones hands over someone actually does something to help them and changes things?

It pivots energy to allow a release and improvement to occur. Yes. Use your hands always when processing a client and not just your ears.

What do you mean by pull things? I sort of know, but only sort of.

In fact, we are pulling blocks, locks, and barriers to well-being and the unfoldment of the soul.

Chapter 16 – Karma Cleansing and Re-Creation

Remember, this work is all about energy. This means re-organization, re-conditioning, re-structuring, re-alignment, re-newel and re-activation of the spirit and body. This means recreation of the being into a raised, enlightened spirit and allowing for a free experience of life on this plane.

Some of us have the awareness that our past-life actions (karma) have an effect on our lives in the here and now. While this may be true, it is also very possible for one to cleanse him or herself of this energy as well as any other ingrained block that might curtail one's delightful experience in the here and now.

Karma cleansing is cleansing of all lifetimes' mis-creations. It is done with the recognition by the client of_ this and all lifetimes' past karmic events and to clear them. The process is simple and can be viewed as past-life regression processing. The principle of not attaching too much importance, either by the client or the practitioner, to what the client finds is the same as in all processes. Just sweep the body and ask for times of actions, omissions, misdeeds, or wrongdoings where the client feels there may be something to clear.

The client can go through a recall process or just allow the practitioner to find whatever he or she might to remove. The practitioner asks for times of concern with karma issues and continues to pull off whatever comes up. Don't be overly concerned with whatever might pop up; the client may be communicating things you'd just as soon not know about. This should not be of any concern to the practitioner as these are generally of the past and in reality may not even belong to the client. That is to say: subjects the client may bring up could, in fact, belong to another person's energy or awareness that somehow the client took on as their own—normally by shifting one's own personality.

Clear Karma cleansing to all points of origin on all topics. To the point of creation, turn polarity, release, and disconnect. Disconnect[19] from ownership; disconnect from attention; disconnect the energy; and the client must be willing to stay disconnected from it. Please help by instructing them to do so.

Be patient and allow everything to come and go, as this is the most effective way to get all that is there. It will require commitment on the part of both the practitioner and the client to work this to completion. The results, however, can be nothing short of miraculous and well worth putting in the time and effort.

Be sure to check all parts of the body when clearing karmic events. As you are not going to be sure where the most charge will be found, be sure to spend ample time with feet, head, and heart Chakra areas.

When this stuff cools down—and it will—end with re-activating the body for re-alignment, re-activation, re-newel, and re-creation.

---

[19]   Disconnection = in order for one to be free, one must disconnect from old habits, thoughts and so on, without the need to re-create that which binds or holds one back from the true destiny — unfoldment.

The client will experience great relief through this process and may go through a series of rather dramatic changes including laughing, crying, or even mild hysteria. Don't be concerned. Just allow the shifts to take place and continue pulling energy while the client is going through his/her changes. Follow with a light, short massage or just a little compassionate handholding.

Dear ones, please excuse my transgressions as I excuse yours. We are just going through a trial and error phase in one lifetime or another. Not to worry, we have Love, Peace and Joy in our hearts now, and NOW is all there is.

* Karma cleansing is the principle of cause and effect and reversal to no effect in the here and now.

Frequently Asked Questions and Answers

Past life? Are you talking reincarnation or do you mean things that have happened to the person in the past?

Past lives and current.

You spoke about the client taking on someone else's "stuff". How does the practitioner keep from taking on the client's negative energies or whatever?

By allowing it to flow out through their crown Chakra and out to other dimensions just by allowing it to flow out without force, or control, or power. By merely allowing it to go elsewhere.

What do you mean by karma?

Cause and effect. The "what we sow we reap" experience. Clean it up and move on.

After the stuff is pulled out of the client, what do I do with it and how?

Send it elsewhere. Send it to a lock box in the desert if you like, but don't attempt to deal with it or clear it. It has a life of its own. Instruct it to find a healing modality so it can find its own unfoldment.

You make it sound as if these things really exist, the same as material things, like a chair for example. Do they?

Unfortunately, yes. They exist. It is part of the game we created.

Chapter 17 – Massage for Babies

A child's body: One of the most beautiful works of humanity and our responsibility is to have, to hold, to cherish, Love and to clear.

It may be true that a practitioner will not find much to clear up on a baby because we tend to come into the world either clear or with lack of much memory or recent trauma. The more that is reactivated, the more undesirable experiences we go through the more there is to clear up. Children of all ages will benefit from regular massage and sweeping of energy blocks in order to calm, align, and raise the child with the highest degree of love and care.

Massage for babies is a very simple, loving process that is doable by any parent or practitioner at any level. The procedure is that of getting started to give a full treatment to an adult.

Rhythmically and evenly touch the body with firm, gentle, loving hands.

Work the entire body. Hold the baby's feet and hands, cupping the head and hold it very gently. Rub the baby's back and tummy softly and smoothly. Work the third eye area in slow motion with even clockwise and counter-clockwise circular movements. Incidentally, this works well for people with ill bodies as well.

As you continue movement of your hands on the body simply pull whatever you perceive that does not feel beneficial to the child. Just keep light touch massage going and flow Love, Peace, and Joy to the child. This is great therapy and a child who experiences this *Gift of Touch* will grow up feeling very loved.

Practice this treatment at times when the child appears to be upset or is crying for no apparent reason. This is by far one of the best ways to help a child relax and fall asleep. You will want to acknowledge the baby's intent to communicate as he or she might be trying to tell you something. You may or may not get an intuitive "hit" for what the baby is saying. It does not matter. Just let the baby know you hear and are there for him/her and continue the process. Pull from the baby being (I know there is no such thing I just like the way it sounds) everything that comes up during the process until it cools down.

Be sure to work the head, face, and neck with very light strokes and loving fingertip touch. The child will respond with a smile or a loving glance into your eyes, or will just fall asleep. The session is then complete.

Children who appear chronically upset may be in need in a change of diet or the removal of one food source or another. Common food allergies are eggs, milk, cheese, wheat, and sugar. If the child appears ill in any way then the parent(s) should consult a physician.

Wonder and Joy babies bring into our lives

Love in the highest order

We see in them as ourselves

The future holds us in Awe

As we gaze into a baby's eyes

Frequently Asked Questions and Answers

What do you mean by "the more that gets reactivated"?

By the more stuff of the mind and cellular memory that is turned on or re-stimulated.

Babies are pretty fragile beings. Is there a chance we could possibly put something in the wrong place by doing this?

No. Touch them with loving kindness and you cannot hurt them.

What do you mean there is no such thing as a "baby being"? Aren't we all beings and wouldn't an infant be considered a baby being?

No. We are all just beings, some younger beings then others perhaps, but no baby beings—sorry.

You said the baby might be trying to communicate something to us. Wouldn't it be easy to figure out what the baby is trying to communicate? I mean, what does a baby know other than being hungry, needing a diaper change, hurting, or maybe be frightened by a loud noise or something?

Ah ye of such little faith. Many clear babies know more than we do.

Chapter 18 – The Sweat Cleansing

A human being has plenty of opportunity to contaminate one's body during a lifetime. The pollutants available seem endless so I'll only mention a handful here. Even with a well-guarded regime of intake it is almost impossible to avoid ingesting or absorbing some materials less then harmonious to our body's materials other then the highest value.

We may seek only high quality, pure water and organic produce but the reality of planet Earth's contaminants could affect us all at one point or another.

I'm talking about products such as chemical fertilizers; hormones added to beef; contaminated milk, eggs, and cheese. Shall I go on? OK! Herbicides, fungicides, pesticides, gas fumes and, of course, impure water, drugs, and alcohol.

While it is true that all of these components make up energy and can be dealt with by the same processes as all other undesirable energy—that is to say, pull it and turn it—there is another avenue one may want to add to one's clearing.

Sweat it out

The Native Americans and Asian people have used sweats for health purposes for thousands of years and been proven effective by science and religious orders.

Sweating, particularly a program of regular sweating requires courage and determination. The practitioner must be able to guide the client through the process and also prepare for a multitude of possibilities that might come up.

The process could involve several days of sweating and ingesting specific herbs and vitamins along with lots of water. For a complete list of herbs and vitamins please refer to Jay North's book titled "Miracles In The Kitchen" available through Jay's website www.OneGlobePress.com . I recommend that anyone considering a long-term sweat consult with a physician before starting.

The temperature of the sweat lodge normally is at the highest degree acceptable to the client. The hotter it is, the more the person sweats, and the quicker the process. Today, the use of a sauna is the most common sweat lodge.

How long does it take to complete a sweat? That is entirely up to the client, practitioner, and health provider. When it feels complete, it is.

The client should be prepared to stay in the sweat lodge for at least several hours and sometimes several consecutive days. It is highly recommended that the client consume large quantities of pure water during this process. It is also important to get on a regime of cleansing herbs and supportive vitamins as the body is going to be pushing a lot of materials out and replacement of vital life force components just might be a good idea.

It is also advisable for the client to work up a good, fast heart rate before entering the lodge to sweat. This could help push undesirable materials even quicker.

For specific herbs and vitamins to ingest during a sweat, consult your professional at the local health food store. Here is just a short list one might consider adding during a sweat: Chaparral, Willow bark, Mugwort, Yellow dock, and Red clover.

One tribe I am very familiar with from the Northwest (the Blackfeet) ingests the herbs in several ways during an initiation. They drink a tea made from the herbs; have an enema with the same herbs; bathe in them; add them to a pot of boiling water during the sweat; and even spank the tribal member with the leaves and branches of the plants they use (sort of like beating the devil out).

Whichever method you choose for clearing the body of unwanted materials, I do encourage you to read one of my books written specifically on the subject of sweats and water purification: *Miracles in the Kitchen, at ww.OneGlobePress.com.* Take it slow; do the programs at a pace that is comfortable; and, as suggested earlier, be sure to consult a health professional before starting what for some people is not an easy process to complete.

The practitioner will want to aid in this program with the client to ensure all is going well but also to encourage the client along the way and to pull and turn as much Energy from the materials as possible—as plenty will surface. Add light or tough massage as required.

NOTE to practitioners and their clients: There is the big possibility that the person doing the sweats is going to experience rather dramatic shifts. This will be most noticeable in personality changes; emotional highs and lows; and in outbursts of communication such as anger, fear, grief, glee, and possibly a display of exhilaration. Most of the time the quick changes one witnesses are temporary and move off quickly. Once more, check with the good doctor before starting a sweat. When the sweat is complete the client will show marked improvement in appearance, attitude, and out-flow of communication.

It is also advisable that the practitioner does the sweats with the client or finds someone who is willing to do it as a team. It is always better for two or more to do this process at the same time. The Northwest Tribe referred to earlier usually has four or more in their ceremonies.

The client should receive massage and energy manipulation during the sweat cleanse or, at the very least, light touching.

Washtae- all is well.

Nature holds many secrets to cleansing and the Native Americans have known of these miracles for centuries.

From Jay's Book Open Spaces:
My Life With Leonard J. Mountain Chief

The Sacred Sweat Lodge

Each one of us has our own experience of miracles preformed in the sweat lodge. Your accounts will be sacred to you one day, and not lightly shared with anyone.

Without revealing any secrets, here is just one of many such accounts of my time in the sacred sweat lodge with Leonard and friends.

Experiences such as this come not nearly often enough

in our lives. You will see and know when you need one, and it is your responsibility to arrange it and seek an accidental miracle. Life will not usually deal you everything you need. It is way too easy to make excuses like, "I don't have time," "It's too hard," or "Where would I find something like that?" But if you are truly seeking the path to fulfillment, freedom from the past, knowledge of yourself, and the answers to life, you will find the time and the meeting place will come. You will make the time, and you will discover that it is time well spent, as I did with Leonard on so many occasions.

"I have a terrible headache, Leonard," I was whining. "This heat is getting to me and I had a massive headache going." It was the hottest August I can remember! In these parts of Montana, we have winter, and we have August; this was one of those years.

Leonard said, "Time for a sweat." In Native life, almost any time is a good time for a sweat, a smoke, a dance, or a chant song.

The sweat lodge is one of the traditional ways of healing mind, body, and soul. Take it quite seriously. As a matter of fact, a person who does not approach it in reverence would not be welcome, nor would a shaman avail himself for treatment and ask one to cross the line to come into the sweat lodge. Crossing the line is a time of reverence for ceremony and one only does this at the right time. A woman must never cross the line during her moon cycle as they consider this very bad luck.

The sweat lodge is similar to the experience of quiet time, only it involves a physical purging in addition to mere reflection. It is a more active pursuit, but produces an after-effect of having been reborn and refreshed. As with the tribal commune, it combines the experience of coming together for self-examination and cleansing of what we have built up in our bodies, hearts, minds, and spirits as we walk through a convoluted world and a time to let go of the world for a short period.

"Time to let go of the world. Let's go into the sweat lodge. Your head problems will be left there," Leonard said.

The sweat lodge of the Blackfeet Nation is a small half dome; one has to kneel to go in. The body of the lodge is made from bent willow and is covered in either canvas or deer hides. Occasionally old rugs are used, but that is not tradition in the Blackfeet Nation.

The lodge usually holds up to six or eight people, but it can be only two if it is a ceremony; sacrifice, or ritual one is setting out to do. River rock is heated to a very high temperature outside the lodge, and in the traditional way a female virgin of the tribe using tree branches, as the rocks must be pure, passes in the rocks. The hot rocks are placed in the center of the lodge and a mixture of water and herbs is poured over them. The opening to the sweat lodge or the door must always face east; there is no other acceptable direction, there is no other way! East represents new beginnings, the sunrise, mother's warmth, and healing.

There is always a leader or a shaman in the lodge, and he directs how the sweat will be run and its designated time. In other words, he decides how long we are to stay in the very dark, very hot lodge. Participants are encouraged to stay in the lodge for the entire duration of the sweat, and not to break the circle. The circle is of supreme importance to the Nation People, and we believe that if the circle had not been broken, we would not have lost our land and sacred buffalo.

The lodge is normally built near cold running water so when it is time to come out, we can dive into a lake or stream. Occasionally the sweat will go on for several days. We enter the lodge as a group and depart together, we take long walks in silence, we rest, we fast, save for water, and we sweat in a harmonious group.

Treatment is often preformed to assist in the overcoming of an ailment, disease, discomfort, or nagging headache, such as the one I went in with.

Physical complaints are not the only reason for a sweat: on the contrary. We sweat to aid in our discovery, we sweat to help elevate ourselves to a place of desired strength and to achieve abilities. We sweat out the devil, we sweat in remembrance and we sweat to clean impurities, both physical and mental, out of our bodies.

Herbs are always used in our sweats, and the ones utilized vary, based on our particular desire and circumstance. Mugwort, willow bark, and chaparral are just a few examples. Herbs are used in many ways and are applied as part of the ceremony. They are breathed in as steam over hot rocks, they are eaten, they are boiled and drunk as tea, they are bathed in, they are taken in through the anus, and they are spanked or beaten into the skin with branches and leaves.

Some herbs make one feel terrible for a short period of time. This is expected. One will experience deep heaves, hot and cold sweats, deep pain and diarrhea. But it all passes and one is encouraged to keep up his courage and allow this process to take place. If you can't, you shouldn't be there in the first place. That is law.

Leonard had gotten word of a ritual sweat about to take place down in the flats at the east end of the Res.

"Come; let us go into the sweat lodge. There is an elder running the lodge today and he will be very happy to see you," Leonard said.

We approached the lower flatlands of Two Medicine River, which twists and turns its way down through what is the desert land off the reservation. Great for fly-fishing, but that was not our purpose this time. When we arrived, I could see about four or five naked old men wandering around a makeshift camp and gathering covers to go over the sweat lodge. The fire was already burning very hot and the rocks were turning white from the coals. The camp was quiet, with the exception of warm greetings when we arrived, and it remained that way. The oldest member of the group, Earl, a small but hugely respected shaman, came over to greet me and said, "Good day for a sweat." He laughed, turned and walked towards the lodge, and signaled for the rest of us to follow. We did, and before I knew it, I was in a very small space with six worldly old gentlemen and the rocks began to come in. I recognized most of the members of the sweat from family gatherings and pow-wows.

Each had a reason for being there, and Earl asked us to state our purpose for being at the lodge that day. He asked each of us not to be concerned with the other members' purpose for their sweat. He said that was his job, and we all laughed out loud. Each man told his story, and each man was allowed to speak completely until done. It was informal, yet guided. We were allowed to pour out whatever we wanted to say and Earl listened and acknowledged us completely. When we had all spoken, Earl started the singing and chanting that we would all follow in and participate with.

Leonard noticed I was tense and asked me to just relax into it and allow whatever was to happen in the sweat lodge to happen, or not. "Try not to expect too much," Leonard said.

Earl had herbs for each of us to ingest. He brought plenty of water for drinking and pouring over the hot rocks. He said he wouldn't let us suffer too much and we could go out for a pee and "what-not" if we wanted to. We were all comfortable, near as I could tell, from the glow of the rocks; faces looked cheerful.

The first seven off twenty eight rocks came in from the door keeper, who also kept the sacred fire going.

Earl then began to move quietly and slowly around the lodge and touch each man. Some replied with a laugh, some with a cry and one with a scream. Earl's movements and touching and caressing went on for what seemed liked several hours. The young lady outside of the lodge continued to send in hot rocks the entire time.

It was extremely hot. Each man washed his face several times with water that was brought in for us. The chanting, praying, and singing went on for several more hours. We were all exhausted and could barely stay awake, which is required. I was starting to fear I would not be able to stand it much longer and thought about a fast move to the door. Every now and then, I could feel Leonard's reassuring hand patting me on the knee as if to say, "its okay, kid, you'll make it."

Suddenly Earl said, "It is done!" We were finished with the sweat and allowed to go outside to cool off.

"Gee, my headache is gone and I feel great," I said. Each man had something to say about the experience that had taken just over forty-eight hours.

What I witnessed in the lodge is very private, but I can tell you this: I saw things you'd think you would never see without the use of hallucinogenic. While the things I saw are secret, they are also very real.

All Leonard had to say was, "Nice sweat, eh? Let's go eat."

One day you will experience a sweat lodge and my prayer and hope for you is that it is traditional and authentic; and that you have someone by your side to pat you on the knee as if to say, "It's okay; you'll make it."

Leonard is gone from his body now, but every now and then I can feel him say, "It's okay Jay, you'll make it."

Frequently Asked Questions and Answers

What do you mean when you say it takes courage and determination to sweat? You get hot, you sweat, isn't that about it? I can see where it could get boring sitting in a sauna for hours at a time, but doesn't sound like it's something that would take braveness especially.

Determination, maybe, but courage?

Some sweats go on for many, many days in a row. It takes courage and determination to stay with it.

What if you don't live where there is a sweat lodge or a sauna available? Is there any kind of a substitute?

NO. Using a native sweat or a sauna is the only way to do this cleansing.

You said something about it taking several hours or even days. What if the sauna isn't open twenty-four hours a day? Do you get there when it opens, stay till it closes and then repeat this the next day and keep on doing this till you feel like something has happened?

Find the schedule that works well for all concerned, but do the sweats. They are vital.

Chapter 19 – Rite of Passage

As it currently appears, we will all drop our bodies eventually and move on. Many great thinkers and writers of this age believe we do so because we believe we will and that with a shift of beliefs, we might go on indefinitely (see the chapter on Cracking the DNA Code, pg. 169). While this may be true for some, let's just assume we will most likely trade up for a somewhat more vital and able body. I do not believe you will ask if this writer believes in reincarnation, as I think that is apparent.

How a being passes on to the next life is of paramount concern and vital interest to this work. We, as practitioners, have the opportunity and for some, the responsibility, to assist the dying in leaving their bodies. Perhaps there is a better term than dying, as there is no such thing as death but merely a passing into a new experience. *"There is only Life, continuous, glorious life. What has been referred to as death is nothing more than releasing a body that no longer serves the needs of the one who owns it."* (White Buffalo Speaks, through Leonard J. Mountain Chief, my adopted father of the great Blackfeet Nation) Or in many cases, the body simply malfunctions and it's time to let it go.

The time of releasing can have an impact on the being's life in its next incarnation and be a contributing factor in how one lives the next life and its outcome. What is important for practitioners to understand is that we have the tools to make leaving the body a somewhat less traumatic event for the person preparing to go off.

Apply this same process when the being is re-entering through rebirth with a new mother.

Whenever possible, try to allow the client leaving an incarnation to leave in a space that is familiar and comfortable.

After goodbyes have been said to friends and family members, if the client has that opportunity, the practitioner should be left alone with the client. This will help facilitate the practitioner's work in assisting in the right of passage treatment-in peace and quiet.

Limit noise and distractions as much as possible: lights low, soft healing music playing. Practitioner flows pure Love, Peace and Joy to the client.

The client is asked to breathe slowly and rhythmically. If the client should start to hyperventilate out of fear of dying, allow him/her to experience it and work to calm the person to an even breathing rate.

The practitioner applies touch to the client; moves around the body and simply touches it. Ask the client, how is it going? Is there anything you would like to say or tell me before you go? Allow what comes up to flow. The client may have a lot to say or very little and this could depend on the person's ability to speak at the time. Allow the client to gesture if that is all he or she will do. Just let the client know you have heard and understand.

As you continue light touch on the body, pull energy off whatever comes up. Do not be concerned what it is. Remember, you are pulling energy and try not to attach too much importance to what is being communicated or what it feels like. Just pull it and send it off.

The person may gradually appear to be calming and settling into acceptance of the "inevitable"; or may struggle a bit, as some of us are not ready to drop the body. For some people this is a scary experience and, for others, quite natural and non-threatening. In any case, continue the work until indications look good or the being passes out of the body or falls asleep to prepare to leave at a later time.

As you prepare to go, know that you are in my heart and we will see one another again.

One gentle old soul I worked with several years ago actually hung around for several days before he decided it was time to let go and take off. Although he had lived a very long and happy life (93 years), he just wasn't ready to let go of an aged, tired, old body that wanted to quit. A couple of times during the night he sat up to talk and then almost instantly would fall back asleep. Then he would awaken to try to catch his breath. He would hyperventilate, swear at the devil and then go back to sleep. We continued to pull energy, wipe his brow, hold onto his feet, and keep a clean space (free of entities), making it as safe and comfortable for him to go as possible. On the fifth day at 4:00 am, he drifted out of the body and his passage was complete.

The rite of passage work can be performed after a being drops the body as well. One can locate the being and do the clearing work that may be required. The effect will still be beneficial to the client. The process is simply to be there for the client; hold parts of their body and sweep and clean energies of whatever comes up. Assist in allowing for a calm passage into the next incarnation.

111

This is extremely rewarding work. There is nothing to fear, as the passing is natural—at least at this juncture—and you are dealing with a being and a body to help free them and reach unfoldment of the soul. If you have not had this opportunity to assist in a passing I suggest looking for the opportunity. The experience will help you in your work immensely.

One-ness in the highest heaven

Allow this soul the rite of Passage to be calm

And light

Great teacher of universal law

Allow this soul to experience

Exactly who it is

We offer you sweet fragrance

And Rose Wine

With these gifts we ask

That passage and

Return is of ease.

Frequently Asked Questions and Answers

What happens after a being passes out of a body because they are through with it? Do they go right into another body? Do they just "hang around" for awhile; and if so, is there a particular waiting place for them to "hang around"?

Both. They (the being) may choose to hang around or just move on, but now that abortion and early death in infants is an issue, bodies are in short supply.

You said that the time of releasing has something to do with the being's next life. Would you explain what you mean by that please?

A being preparing to leave his/her body could be in a state of mind of asking what is next and may not choose to go until he/she has made up its mind.

Rite of passage sounds more like what happens when a child becomes, or is considered to have become, an adult. Do you feel that there is some sort of similarity here?

No. This is specific to help the dying make the passage into the next incarnation.

Chapter 20 – On Love…

"When Men and Women can have peace and compassion, there will be Love" Thich Nhat Hahn

The subject of romantic love has baffled many of history's Magi as well as our brightest contemporary thinkers. No one can lay claim to having it all figured out. Love and relationships have confused us for as long as there has been the concept of coupling.

Somehow we have caused the destruction of Love that has existed for millions of years. Can the cycle be broken/changed and re-created into the persistence of Love without the need for destruction or re-creation? The question is: Can Man/Woman love completely and unconditionally, without the need for separation from One-ness? Can we make it through the maze of projections, conclusions, barriers, judgments, fears, postulates, and love/hate opposition without the necessity to counter-create (the destruction of love)— once Love is created?

Can Man/Woman find a way to couple and become conscious enough to move through life with clean hands and a clean heart? In other words, can we learn to walk the straight and narrow, without committing harmful acts on one another that ultimately destroy a partnership?

When we commit harmful acts, it matters—whether or not we consider our actions harmful, helpful, constructive, or destructive. Polarity can be good or bad, negative or positive, and will determine the time span of the union. This depends on whether whomever in the union committed or omitted an act (good or bad) considered to be harmful can or will and does not withhold the fact they did something they consider harmful.

It is actually the withholding that creates the separation.

These are all interesting points of view no doubt, and I'm sure you'll want to turn polarity on each. This is the stuff karma considerations are made of, and they assist in creating closeness or separation in a partnership. They will add to the creation of love or take one through the destruction of the coupling.

Only we determine how our relationships will sail—smoothly or over rocks—by our actions and by our thoughts and words. It is indeed the *thoughts, words, actions, and vibrations* that we create that will ultimately guide our love life—and, of course, our desire to have long-lasting relationships or marriages in the first place.

And then there is the *consideration* of *agreements, definitions, postulates* and future *mock-ups* that can also impact the viability of a union. When two people stick to the original postulate; growth creations and future hopes and dreams mock-ups; their relationship stands a better chance of longevity than those who play it by ear day-to-day. Yet another interesting point of view, I am sure.

Can Man/Woman Love completely and unconditionally within the continuum of love without a counter survival postulate or a destructive postulate or force impinging on the creation of love? In other words, can we love completely and forever, without time, space, or matter having an effect on our ability to love?

Yes! We can, provided we can positively process the negative elements that create separation and devour love.

It has been postulated by the greatest thinkers of all time—including all that we have ever read, met, or heard of in recent years—that Love reigns supreme. There is no higher power then love and all we have to be is Love. As a matter of fact, there is neither doingness nor havingness to love. Only Being. We can create the attribute of love and flow love out into the world without the need to have it return—or do anything for that matter—and be completely fulfilled in our own lives simply from the act of emanating Love by flowing Love out into the world or flowing love to a specific point or terminal. This flowing of love practiced conscientiously and consciously on a continual basis, can bring significant change to planet Earth on many levels and/or dimensions.

Other factors that can have a contributing effect on the longevity of Love relationships are 1) Communication and 2) Problem solving.

A well-known author (who shall remain nameless) once remarked that, "communication is the universal solvent," and that every situation can be handled by communicating effectively. The willingness and ability to communicate are definitely attributes on which all couples can improve. It takes guts sometimes; particularly when one is hiding emotionally; but it is indeed true that communication is the universal solvent. Why is that you ask? Because there is not a problem in the world that cannot be handled by communication. It defies the laws of physics to think there is. Even tribal wars could be ended this way.

Communication and Forgiveness handles all ills. It is essential that barriers to communication and problem solving are processed till non-existent. Turn polarity on all inability to love unconditionally. Draw back your power and watch your love grow.

The other important factor is problem solving. It goes right along with the communication equation. What is a problem but two aspects of the same issue with opposing points of view which generally contain equal magnitude? The ability to solve problems simply comes from one's willingness to look at the problem; to spot the opposing points of view; and to postulate a conclusion. And turn polarity to a point there is no charge on what was once a problem.

When there is love then both factors are in place: the ability to communicate and the ability to see and solve problems. A couple should do this naturally. Where there are blocks, in all cases: run interesting point of view; turn polarity. It is simply a matter of the creation and practice and out-flowing of Love in the present moment of now that creates Love in the now and into forever.

It is not a matter of Create, Survive, and End. It has everything to do with the planet Earth postulate of Start – Change – Stop. There is Create and Destroy game; there is Love created in the present moment of now— and on a continuum of nowness and an end creation or destruction.

The process to undo the mock-up of Love ending or Love destruction is to have the client open the heart Chakra and go completely into Love allowance.

You, the practitioner, sweep the body for blockages that

disallow Love from being persistent. Check for polarities and use your intuition to find blocks. Pay particular attention to the heart and third eye Chakras, root Chakra and solar plexus.

- Run point of creation; turn polarity processes throughout the entire session.

- Turn polarity on all definitions of Love throughout all time, all space, and dimensions.

- Turn polarity on the history of love, get the stuck to postulate.

- Turn polarity, just as a reminder is to pivot the energy, dissipates the charge; there by setting the soul free.

Runs like this: on the subject of Love all counter-thoughts, postulates, ideas, considerations, projections, judgments, conclusions, agreements; on the subject of the Creation of Love being throughout all time, all space, and all dimensions: turn polarity, release and disconnect. Run each item separately and completely to point of creation and turn polarity on each. Sweep the entire body, paying close attention to the root, heart, and third eye; pull blocks from wherever shows up, including the root and heart Chakras. Find entities that may have an opinion, turn polarity, and ask the entity to release.

Find with and for your client all impediments (blocks) on or to Love, throughout all time and all space and all dimensions; get all fingers, all maps, all weight, mass, glops, *FEELINGS,* mechanisms, hidden in the heart, agreements that hold in place the thought-idea of Love *destruction. You can find and turn polarity on as much of this stuff as possible,* 'cause, folks, this is the stuff that will change the planet.

- Get the Love/hate syndrome postulates.

- Get all contracts to disconnect postulates.

- Check for all fears (big common barrier).

- Run (pull) all can't-have-must-have Love.

- Clean off postulate to not allow self to Love again.

- Clean the cycle of Create-Survive-Destroy on Love.

- Get the Died-for-Love postulate.

- Find the must-have/can't-have decisions on love; turn polarity and all thoughts just prior to the point of creation. Turn polarity; release, and disconnect.

- Check the feet, the head, and the hands for the Game of Love or Love as a Game postulate.

- Clean all the above running points of creation; turn polarity, all space, all time, all dimensions; get the weight, mass motion, all sensations, and continuum to not allow Love as a viable presence in the here and now, release and disconnect.

- Get the thought prior to the point of creation of

love destruction and turn polarity.

- Turn all postulates in relation to contracts counter to the survival of Love. Turn polarity; release, and disconnect.

- Find the make-wrong postulate on women and men that creates further separation.

- Ask for the evildoer's postulate that creates the I-gotta-get-out-of-here syndrome; (this is created by the concept of karma). Turn polarity; release, and disconnect.

- Turn polarity on all the decisions to hate one 's self, Can't Love Self, Must Love Self, Stuck on Self, Therefore Can't Love Others.

- Find willingness/non-willingness to love; turn polarity, release, and disconnect.

Sweep as long as it takes, and try to get all of this done and over within one session—although this is a pretty hot area so you may have to count on more than one session.

Bring the client to the point of willingness in this zone of now-willing-to-set-a-new-postulate to guide the future of his/her willingness to love.

I, (Client Name), do hereby rescind, renounce, recall, recount and reject all contracts, vows, promises and postulates to end, stop, and/or destroy love. There is no re-creation to love; there is only love creation.

By turning polarity, you, the practitioner, are decreasing the amount of charge and impact on your client from a whole host of impingements. Turning polarity is changing a thing from negative to positive until your client reaches realizations. Turn polarity by feelings, not thought. Just give instructions to turn and allow whatever **IT** is to do so.

You find postulates the same way: ask for the postulates and allow them to come up; pull 'em and turn 'em.

End session with head manipulation or light massage at the top of head and cover all scalp area. Turn on; call up re-creation, re-activation and re-alignment.

Yes, it's OK to let go of relationships; for beings to go off in their own directions (there is no separation), the only thing is, love will still be there. Why? Because, just like life, one cannot destroy love.

If we focus our thoughts on all that is good and kind and beautiful we shall see God's love in spite of all the ugliness that exists in human nature Hazrat Inayat Khan ("interesting point of view, turn polarity").

Frequently Asked Questions and Answers

When you speak of turning polarity, it sort of makes me think of a magnet. While we ordinarily think of it as attracting things, it can also reject them. Is this the same sort of thing?

Turning polarity is just that. We ask a thing to pivot enough to allow charge to dissipate and by doing so we become clear and free.

You said that one can not destroy love. If someone is cruel to someone, such as in an abusive situation or marriage, can't the abuse destroy love?

No. Forgive them, move on, and love remains intact.

What do you mean by disconnect? It sort of sounds like unplugging something.

Yes. Exactly. Unplug and let it go, release and disconnect.

Chapter 21 – Clearing the Body, Cells, Aura, and Being of Blocks, Charges and Polarities

It is fairly well recognized today that the body and the beingness of an individual contain charges and polarities on a cellular level that exist in and around the human form. And these electrically charged polarities could impinge or aid one's everyday quality of survival and experience on this planet.

In fact, all thoughts, ideas, conclusions, considerations, agreements, judgments, projections, desires, needs, wants and a whole host of negative concepts and emotions including fear, anger, grief and so on, possess (have) the element of polarity (positive and negative forces) that are in fact a lie! Why? Because thoughts that create the illusion of separation, discomfort, pain, dis-ease and anything other than perfection are all lies. We are, in fact, perfect.

As native beings, we are all perfect.

Polarities can be changed, charges dissipated, and conditions completely improved and a being returned to a fully vibrant level of experience on this plane. How? Simply by instructing it, (energy) to do so, it shall. Ask charge to turn polarity and it will. There is no need for force or effort; without creating a need for an arduous experience, just tell whatever the polarity is to turn and allow it to do so. Trust and have faith that what you are doing is important—because this stuff works, folks. Yes, have fun with the work, but do not take it too lightly or as a joke. It is not. You can indeed help to change an individual life, which no other facilitation (modality) has even a close chance of doing. Sorry if that sounds offensive to some practitioners; it's just that I know what this work can do and you will come to find this is so as well.

We live on a polarized planet (universe) in a polarized and dense society and bodies. Polarization looks and feels like hot and cold, black and white, green and red, yellow and purple, heavy and light, bad and good, evil and kindness and so on. You will know this stuff when you work (feel) it. You already know everything there is to know, so you already know what this stuff feels like. Never underestimate your ability to *know*. It is much the same as when you hear a lie, you just know it's a lie. You can even hold this stuff in your own hands and ask what it is.

Try not to make this heavy work

Please try your very best to not attach too much importance to what you read, hear or see, especially on TV or in the news. Take it all as just an interesting point of view. This work is about getting people unstuck from (mass) heaviness, considerations, not adding to them. We have created this form of processing with a limited amount of form and structure. We are working to decrease the charge of group thought and opinion and the influence of TV-sponsored solidity and to decrease form and structure[20], not add to it.

In our enlightenment, we shall all lighten up and become less in order to have more or nothing at all.

---

[20]   Form and structure = solidity, solidity = more mass, more mass = less fun.

As with all procedures, when doing this work, we turn polarity[21] on the point of creation of the *item* we are working on or with. We release and disconnect from the force that tied our attention to the thing to begin with; i.e., "apples make me feel ill." Hmm, interesting point of view. Turn polarity. On the thought just prior to the creation of *apples make me feel ill,* turn polarity.

Allow it to turn; no force, there are no prayers that will be necessary; just allowance, and sha-bang! It turns and the consideration/condition is gone. This is ancient stuff and nothing new, just written in a form that may be somewhat new.

By the way, yes, you are using your hands the entire time to locate the charge in/on the body for/with your client, and you are pulling the charge at the same time you are asking it to turn. You, the facilitator/practitioner, are pulling, directing, and out-flowing all at the same time. It's not hard; it's not tricky, and, yes, a child can and has done this work! When you pull this stuff and are directing energies to turn polarity, OPEN your crown Chakra and release every bit of the energy blocks and so on as you pull, allow nothing to stick on/in you. Tell this stuff to go and it will. Send it to a lock box in the dessert or the pyramids in Egypt; just send if off to another dimension. And do not worry about processing energies that you release for your client. If you find that you have released an entity (or two), provide instructions for it (them) to find a healing modality that will allow for its own enhanced existence

---

21 Turn polarity, throughout all time and all space in all dimensions, turn polarity on *apples make me feel sick;* turn polarity, release and disconnect.

and survival on whatever plane of its choice.

You will feel the vibration of the charge as you are pulling and directing. You will know that the charge has released and disappeared by the way it feels, by how the client looks, and by what they say. Sometimes the effect will be slight; other times it will be dramatic. End every session with simple scalp manipulation. Activate re-creation, re-activation and re-alignment.

There is a whole host of blocks that can be relieved simply by working the scalp, a subject we are about to cover completely.

Turn polarity on all unwanted conditions, sensations, thoughts, ideas, consideration, conclusions, decisions, fears, doubts, reservations, agreements to suffer, counter production judgments, and projections.

May hands be blessed that know the work that has led to their freedom.

Frequently Asked Questions and Answers

Do you mean you are using your hands to remove these blocks?

Yes, you are using your hands to sweep over the client's body, to spot (feel) the charge. In fact, you are using your hands and intention to facilitate the shifting, manipulation and ultimate removal of unwanted charges (energies). It works like this: open your crown Chakra; pull stuff off your client; blow it out through your crown Chakra to wherever you like. (Please don't attempt to handle or deal with energies removed. It takes too much time and effort and produces very little.) Simply release pulled stuff to another dimension or send it to a lock box in the desert. Continue to send it off, allowing nothing to resonate or stick to you. If you notice a shift in your personal environment (body, personality and so on) pull it and send it off as well. Yes, now and then you will pull off an entity that desires and requires processing; it's up to you process or not.

Electrically charged stuff in and around our bodies that actually have an influence on our survival? Do you mean real electricity like we get when we plug something in?

I am referring to cellular electrical energy in and around the body and have been measured by contemporary science many times in many ways. Now, you can FEEL it, grab hold of it, and turn it until it dissipates and goes away. I e; locks, blocks and barriers,

All stuff like grief and pain and the unpleasant things don't exist? They are a lie and we are perfect? But it seems to me that they exist as much as the pleasant things, we just don't like them. I must be missing something here. Would you explain what you mean please?

Yes we humanoids need a game to play, we need to trick ourselves into thinking we need to figure something out, when in reality we know everything, we are perfect and as in the I Am we are. And so it is. Until we come to this realization, turning polarity is essential.

Chapter 22 – Use Your Head to Change Your Life

According to my information, that I get or receive, the head contains many blocks that are rather common to all people. It seems as if the head has been involved in a huge conspiracy or agreement to hold, hide and contain blocks, locks, barriers, and implants. Secrets that once exposed will, or at least may, lead to man/woman's freedom and wholeness beyond what heretofore has been recognized as possible, important, and vital to the relief of human suffering and from the condition of bondage. (Bondage, in this sense, relates to the common factor of entrapment to conditions and elements of life that we judge as not fun, light, or easy to experience.)

The practitioner/facilitator can move/remove a lot of stuff for the client simply by working the head completely. There are thirty-six points on the head, down the neck and at the occipitals that contain and hold a lot of charge, blocks and all other "stuff", and when pulled and relieved can create a rather interesting change in your client's life. (And in yours for that matter, I do hope you plan to get this work done for yourself as well.) One pulls these energies, blocks and considerations by becoming a vacuum, by allowing your body to be an instrument to move and remove. Simply by feeling the energies, pulling them and blowing them off through your crown Chakra you will assist your clients to lighten their load considerably.

Starting at the forehead or the brow, pull[22]. This

---

[22] Pull = to remove

headwork always requires pulling; i.e., on all points all over the head you will be pulling off energies and blocks and releasing this stuff to wherever!

Just over the eyes, pull Sadness and Joy.

Just above the eyes, pull Considerations of Time and Space.

Pull all points until they cool off.

Work both sides of the head and around the ears, starting behind the ear and working upwards. Starting low, work Kindness, Gratitude, Peace and Calm.

Work up to just over the top of the ear; pulling Creating Connections and Creating Life Forms and Control.

Working now just over the ears and in front of them, pull Money, Awareness, and Communication.

Just at the temples, work in front of the ears and pull Form and Structure, Healing and Hopes, and Dreams.

At the front of the head in the center between the eyes, on the third eye and at the back of the head, at the same time pull Power.

Just above that to the right and left under the ear, pull Implants.

On top of the head, just over the eyes at the normal hairline lay out as lines or cigars, pull Body and Sexuality, Thoughts, Ideas and Considerations.

From out on the sides to the center: Bridging, Aging, Re-creation, Re-activation, Re-alignment and Re-newel, at the center just over the crown, the Circle of Mystery.

And at the crown Chakra- Manifestation.

You are working these areas to remove blocked energy so that the client opens up to experiencing these joyous elements in life. Remove blocks to allow one to experience the joy without negative charge being a factor.

When you work these areas work as slowly or as quickly as required, but pull each area until it cools or energy stops flowing freely. This manipulation can go on for lifetimes to come. No rush, right? It took billions of years to get into this mess, so are you in a big rush to solve it all in a day? Probably won't happen — at least not yet.

At the end of this process, you run you hands over the entire body to re-align, four inch above the client's body, balance the Chakras and get an even energy flow going. When the client shows marked improvement, end the session.

You will be working with these points a lot during sessions, and especially working re-creation, re-activation and re-alignment after each session with your client. This helps to start fresh our new experience after each session and create a new reality to begin anew.

While these points may appear at the outset to be a little odd, it is known that pulling the blocks from these areas on the head will create a dramatic improvement in your client's life, and yours, when you learn to solo process your own stuff off. You should instruct clients how to manipulate these areas themselves, as this work is a process and will require more than one session. Clients can get these points working simply by calling them up. It works like this: The client touches the point he or she wishes to activate and says aloud, *I am* for instance, *I am healing; I am money; I am creating life forms,* etc. The more often you work the points, the quicker the charge will come off and the faster positive changes will come.

Please don't discount the value of working these points on the head, as the improved condition for your client can be rather dramatic. I have personally experienced rather interesting sudden changes in my client's lives with just one of these sessions.

We can, in fact, live in harmony, experiencing peace, joy and glory in abundance.

Frequently Asked Questions and Answers

A lot of those things you talk about pulling sound like good things, love, peace, etc. Why would you want to remove good things?

They are good things and we are not pulling off good stuff, we are pulling blocks off, just by calling it up and asking it to turn polarity, and then we come into the wholeness experience and joy.

You mention that it took billions of years to get into this mess. Does that mean that you think that we are billions of years old?

Yes we are!

Do you think that we are all the same age and started out together or are new beings coming into existence at different times?

We all know one another!

Do we ever reach the point where we don't come back?

This is by choice.

When you say, "pull all points until they cool off", what do you mean by cooling off?

There is no charge left, no vibration, no pull or heaviness, it has cooled off and it is finished leave it alone.

You speak of pulling specific things from specific parts of the body. Does that mean that there are parts of the body where these things are located and that they are the same in everyone?

Yes, it is something we have in common.

Chapter 23 – The Agreement to Suffer

A major factor in suffering — our agreement to do so...

One might ask, "Why in the world would I make an agreement to suffer for another person throughout all time, all space, and all dimensions?" Why would you make such an agreement? Because, dear ones, we are so loving, so good, so compassionate, and the thought of another sentient being suffering upsets us so much that it is beyond our capability to handle. We would rather actually do the suffering ourselves and suffer in place of our friend, lover, or comrade. We would rather and do **now** suffer for one. This is a way pre-Buddha concept. Except that it just doesn't really work. Why? Because it kills oneself!

Apparently, some six billion years ago we all became part of a universal agreement (Universal Surrogate) to join a brother/sisterhood of suffering for one another. Yes, we were all part of the agreement somewhere on our life track; some just demonstrate the implant more than others. In all cases, you should pull this off your client's case (sooner rather than later).

Note to practitioners: Have this pulled from your own Beingness as well

It works something like this: I love you so much; I am your brother/sister. I will not allow you to suffer. I take your Suffering, Pain, Discomfort, Dis-ease, Wrong Doing, and Wrong Thinking from you and now suffer in your place. Great arrangement if you like death, pain, and suffering.

Folks, this is one you gotta go for right away with your clients. Get it turned and pull it. This, in fact, will relieve a lot of suffering your client is experiencing now in this time and space dimension.

Get all willingness to suffer for; do point of creation; turn polarity, release and disconnect throughout the process to pull the charge off this agreement.

This procedure will take off victim charge and will allow the client to return to his or her own power.

Let's go after this Universal Surrogate to suffering; see if we can get it pulled, turned and release us to live in Oneness without the need of separation of the sexes. *Also, part of this program the need for men and woman to have an opponent!*

Start with the head; pull blocks connected to power at the third eye Chakra and occipital; pull until these areas cool.

Pull energy from the feet, the hands and the base of the neck. Pull from the crown Chakra; balance the Chakras throughout the body. Pull energy from the crown Chakra down through the client's palms.

Sweep your hands over the client's body; call up the Universal Surrogate to suffering, ask for all agreements throughout all time, all space, and all dimensions. Get all incidents of agreeing to suffer for another. **Get to the Core**.

Please don't make a big deal of time, place, events, and so on. We are just after the energy connected to time, space, and matter; don't hang yourself up on the importance of specifics. Just turn the polarity (energy); get it all at the original points of creation and turn it.

Get the point of creation of the thought just prior to point of creation of the agreement itself; turn polarity, release, and disconnect.

Ask for brotherhood/sisterhood to the alignment, agreement to suffer for another, turn polarity, release and disconnect.

Ask for, I'll-step-in-for-you (individual, group or nation) to suffer for; turn polarity.

Pull the guardian to the gate of suffering; pull Christ connected to suffering for; pull the benevolence to suffering for; find the enlightened ones that agree to suffer for; release them and send them off to a healing modality.

Turn the willingness to suffer for Oneness throughout all time, all space, and all dimensions, turn polarity, release and disconnect.

Locate all Implants inserted, reinforced and held in place; the agreements, willingness/unwillingness, resistances or postulates related to will, can't-suffer to suffering-for; PIVOT, turn polarity on each.

Next, check for any secret society, undercover, covert, hidden, covered-up, lied-about, denied agreements, and willingness to suffer.

Go to the point of creation on all manifestations, creations, postulates, considerations, conclusions, decisions, convex, concave, fixations, truths, untruths, willingness, agreements to suffer for; turn polarity throughout all time, all space, and all dimensions; turn polarity; release and disconnect. Ask client to draw back their personal power and live free of suffering in the here and now.

End off with this: On the head, pull energy, re-structuring, re-activation, re-creation.

Have the client recount, recall, rescind, revoke, and remove all agreements, conclusions to suffer in this time/space experience: *I, _____, send all energy to suffering, all agreements to Universal Surrogate to suffering, off to a place of non-existence, to a dimension of powerlessness, neither control nor power in this dimension on individual it's connected to suffering for. I live a life free of suffering.*

End with gentle sweep of the body to realign all of the Chakras.

Hold feet in hands for a few moments. End session.

Release this stuff from your own personal environment (body) by blowing this charge off and out through your crown Chakra.

According to the contemporary Zen Master Thich Nhat Hahn, we are, in fact, responsible to heal the suffering of all sentient beings, just don't allow it to stick with you.

Frequently Asked Questions and Answers

Six billion years old? Where did you get this information? You make it sound like you know what you're talking about.

Thank you, I do. It came to me, please go back to the beginning of the book, and see acknowledgements.

If we made an agreement like this, and have been experiencing someone else's suffering, will someone else start suffering if it is pulled off from us?

No, we have relieved the suffering and sent this energy elsewhere.

Do we always reincarnate with the same group of people?

Could be, this is a matter of choice. Personally, I have lived all over the globe and on many planets and have known many people for billions of years and so have you.

Chapter 24 – Forgiveness

There is much forgiveness for the seeker of truth. When one opens their heart to forgiveness then miracles occur easily, effortlessly and naturally.

One is asked to let down all defenses, all blocks and the need to be right, forgive, and allow great healing to occur...

The effects of one forgiving another, and one's self are among the highest achieved goals in healing. One will experience a re-vitalized spirit, healthier body, renewed love for one's self and all other living things. Experience the achievement of spiritual elevation through forgiveness.

Process yourself and your client up through mistaken un-forgiveness and come out flying like an eagle. Come into sacred forgiveness and experience your own miracles.

Excerpt from Open Spaces: *My Life and Times* with
Leonard J. Mountain Chief

Leonard and I often took long, slow walks in the hills around Heart Butte Montana. As we walked, he loved to tell Indian stories of long ago. Often he would start them with, "When the grass was knee high..."

Leonard saw, as many of us do, too much needless suffering. One day while we were walking, he spoke of forgiveness.

"When we look around the world today, we find much needless suffering," he said. "The causes are indeed vast. People everywhere are hurt, lonely, and depressed. Some are just starving for a simple hug."

He went on to say that people's lives could be changed and improved through the simple act of forgiveness. "While this may be a foreign concept for some," he said, "it will be easy for others to grasp and apply to their lives, to help promote a new outlook and experience.

"I hope you will see the value of forgiveness in your life," he said. "I believe that people can understand that they can actually be free, simply through the act of forgiveness. Recall Christ's words on the cross, 'Forgive them, Father, for they know not what they do.' Christ's love for all humanity was so strong, that even in his own deep suffering all he could consider was forgiveness."

"Native people have been confronting this subject and dealing with issues connected to forgiveness for many years," said Leonard. "We can choose to excuse or forgive our enemies, so called evil ones, spouses for wrongdoings or mistakes made against us, however perceived. We can forgive our neighbors and live in peace.

"There is no doubt that there is a world of hurt all around us," he went on. "As each and every person, group and clan has some perceived vision of being wronged, we can feel victimized occasionally by those who wish to oppress us in one way or another. Throughout history, for many thousands of years, people have felt taken advantage of, hurt, used, and abused. It goes beyond feelings. It touches on our core of beliefs, emotions, and the very basic trusts we have in people around us. Many people feel somehow betrayed.

"But what if, just perhaps, our own experience can be made more pleasurable by forgiveness? What if it can become easier to get along, live well, and prosper beyond our current circumstance if we can learn to forgive? What if this is possible?"

Referring to the tribe's hatred of Whites, Leonard said, "If we can learn to forgive the White man, we'll all be better off. It is time for us to forgive and move on."

"But Leonard," I asked, "How can you tell me to forgive someone who has done me a horrible wrong? What if this person murdered my child or raped me or cheated my family out of our money?"

"Forgive them," he said.

This heartfelt conversation with Leonard brought to mind an incident at a concert in Los Angeles that my beautiful African-American then girlfriend and I were attending. The concert was intended primarily for an African-American audience, and a young man approached my companion and asked her, "What are you doing with this honky"?" We were holding hands.

I stepped in to answer for her, "Look man, I'm not a honky any more than you are a Negro. If you cut me, you will see I am exactly like you. And if you are cut, you will see you are exactly like me. We will both bleed. We are the same. We both appreciate a beautiful woman, it's time we forgive one another's race and move on, for we are, in fact, brothers."

He stood silent for a moment, laughed, and agreed.

We hugged and that was the last I saw of him, and no other negative events happened that night.

Leonard said, "We Homo Sapiens can find all sorts of supposedly justifiable reasons to hate one another. Out of fear-based conclusions that create our barriers, we have held on to the separation instead of actually loving one another and realizing our Oneness in The Great Spirit.

"The lack of forgiving rarely harms the person one refuses to forgive. Harm comes to the one who refuses to forgive. Hatred, bitterness, and grudges eat away at the soul of one holding them inside," said Leonard.

"What many fail to realize about forgiveness is that if the person deserves to be forgiven, it isn't forgiveness! Forgiveness is a unique act reserved for those who have harmed us, either intentionally or unintentionally, and who do not deserve forgiveness for their actions.

"When we are wronged," he said, "we have a choice: to forgive or not to forgive. Forgiving, truly forgiving, is difficult. We must surrender our right to hold a wrong against an offender. It defies our human need to defend ourselves and avenge ourselves."

He went on, "The alternative is un-forgiveness. Let's take a look at that decision. When we fail to forgive our offenders, we hold something harmful within ourselves. This ugly thing isn't in them—it is in us. We carry it. We become frustrated, because we see the person who has done us wrong, and they seem fine. They are happy and going about their business while we, the offended, are often ill and miserable.

"Frustration leads, as any psychologist will tell you, to

141

anger. Anger causes further harm to others, who in turn confront the decision to forgive or not to forgive, or to turn it inward. Do you know what psychologists call, "anger turned inward"? Depression!" he said.

"I know of no human, male or female, black, white, red, or brown, young or old, rich or poor, who has never been wronged. Every one of us will face the decision to forgive at some point in our lives—and most of us will face it many times over. Will we forgive, releasing our offender—but more—releasing ourselves from the bondage of hatred? Or, will we become frustrated, angry, depressed, or lash out and leave a fresh trail of hurt across humankind?

"Forgiving is hard. It requires us to let go of our right to avenge those who have hurt us. The alternative is easier, but vastly more destructive," said Leonard.

"But not all is hopeless," Leonard continued. "If we decide and if we choose, we can evolve through this appearance of a downward spiral of fear-based hatred and come out stronger, happier, and healthier. We can live in peace with all people everywhere as one in the Great Spirit.

"Oh sure, the skeptics are saying, you can never put two opposing groups or tribes in a room and ask them to forgive each other. You cannot bring peoples together that have hated one another for centuries and say, 'Okay, guys, now it's time to love each other,' but I beg to differ," said Leonard. "What would life be like if we simply said, 'I forgive you? I love you. You are my brother or my sister and I wish for the fighting, dying and starvation to end. Can we please forgive one another and move on?'

142

"Just as an example," he said, "let's try this: I forgive the police for pretending to be Nazis. I forgive armies for the killing of innocent women and children. I forgive the government for acts of treason. I forgive corporations for taking advantage of less-educated people in Third World countries and starving their children. I forgive the Whites for suppressing Blacks, Hispanics, Natives, and Asians for hundreds of years. I forgive my spouse for debasing me. I forgive the rapist who took my life from me. I forgive my parents for not wanting me and not understanding how to raise a child. I forgive the teachers in my school that understood little more than control. I forgive my farther for raping my sister and beating my brothers and me on a daily basis. I forgive all those who have falsely accused me and attempted to damage my reputation.

"And while you're at it, one could say, 'I forgive myself for all the wrongdoings I have committed throughout all of my life to everyone, everywhere.' One could even say a short prayer and ask for forgiveness for the acts of violence or acts of omission one has committed in his or her own life experience towards all other people, animals, plants and trees."

"Whoops," he said, "that means taking responsibility seriously, now, doesn't it?"

"And what's the outcome we might expect? Well, why don't we all just do a little experiment starting today and find out? Find someone to forgive. Let them know you forgive them and ask them to forgive one other person. Look at it this way, what is there to lose? Your pride? Your manhood? Your woman's integrity? Nothing at all should stand in the way of the peace we could experience through forgivingness. If three people forgive three people and they forgive three others, there is no telling where it might lead." "To World Peace?" He asked.

Leonard said, "There is no higher purpose than love and if we can do this simple act we can, in fact, live in our highest and best realization of ourselves." There is no other way, he said.

"I'll start today, and why don't you join me? If you don't," he said, "I forgive you."

The Process to un-forgiveness

Process one through the inability to forgive, the client will come out "clean" and or no charge on people once disliked. Client will regain ability to take responsibility for one's own life.

Turn polarity on all items containing un-forgiveness.

Run client through each as follows:

Can't forgive

Unwilling to forgive

Won't be forgiven

Too much hate to forgive

That so and so did to me

I just can't forgive him or her

No, to heavy I just can't forgive

144

They are too stupid to be forgiven

There are just some things that can't be forgiven

God can forgive that but not me

Oh, I can never be forgiven for what I have done

Find back up hidden inability to forgive

Find black spots to aid in un-forgiveness

Find and remove walls to forgiveness

Are you kidding me, he/she ruined me I can't forgive them

Never. I will never forgive what he/she did to me

Get all shame, blame and regret on this item

Run all this lifetime deeds one needs to forgive one's self for

Run all past life deeds, acts, and omissions on others, asking for forgiveness

Find all resistance to forgiveness

Find all agreements to not forgive

Pull group agreements to un-forgiveness

Ask the client to come up with all un-forgiveness they can spot holding on in place

As in all processes, use point of creation, turn polarity, turn polarity throughout all time, all space, all dimensions, release and disconnect. If client feels like they are holding on to un-forgiveness—that is, you feel it in them, not them feeling it per se. * Rerun all the above till clear.

End off with re-activation, re-alignment, and re-newel

Ask client to sit quietly in nature—even a park for the rest of the day. You can gain much from this process so don't discount its effectiveness. Allow your client and self to experience the wondrous joy by drawing back the power lost through mistaken un-forgiveness.

Chapter 25 – The Origins of Traps

The number-one, major origin of traps is the **mind**; as I said before, get rid of it (the mind) and you'll be a lot better off. "The Mind Is a Wonderful Thing to Waste", which could be a great title for my next book.

Mental traps

Traps we have been taught, created, resisted, accepted or agreed to all do the same thing: they lock us **in** and hold us back, make less of our beingness and our ability to create what we desire most on this plane: Love, Peace, Joy, Freedom and Prosperity. Traps, barriers, blocks and self-created walls and boxes, all created, agreed upon and/or tied to, resisted; the one thing they have in common is they tend to hold us down and in place, and the mind is responsible. Not unlike world Governments of history, in some cases contemporary. But no victims here, right?

The only real power (mind) traps have is the energy we give them. We can, in fact, simply rise above them all and be our natural God/Goddess-hood-selves and in control of our personal knowingness and power.

This work comes from years of observation and practice. While I would like to give credit to all of the contemporary original teachings, because of various church rules, copyright laws of others and dumb stuff like that, in some cases (not all), I cannot give credit where credit is due! Know this my friends: I bring you this work of my own knowingness and experience and with the aid of few special guides.

I will offer this note however: Now, in this time, form,

dimension, these writings come to me from sources or entities outside of this plane. I do not claim to be a channel that brings messages that you do not already have access to. I am simply bringing forth ideas that will facilitate one's own healing and movement towards Oneness and the final destination.

And what does Oneness offer? Everything from the heavens desired on this plane.

With that said, I will now run through rather quickly and briefly some entrapments or fields of considerations that may, and probably do, hold one in or fixated to, a not so pleasurable experience.

Not in any particular order that you will have to run, but I would check for these items on your client (and yourself, as well of course.).

Traps we have adequately created for ourselves

Trap #1: For not helping me, you so-and-so!

This is so typical, and it's amazing how often it goes unnoticed. The need people have for making one another wrong! Why is that, you may ask? Yes, and well you might! Excellent question, considering that making one wrong is so prevalent in our world today we actually fight wars because of it- and how unnoticed it goes.

The make-wrong and built-in need to attack the helper

148

comes from the same, or at least very similar, implanted postulate common to many people, the mind! Its origination is from very long ago, it contains automatic instructions to make self-right, and all others wrong— and attack anyone who offers aid, assistance or HELP.

When we find ourselves so frustrated, we are unable to communicate at all. Wracked with problems, facing disasters at every turn: home, country, workplace, loss of personal power and needless restrictions on our activities—and, God knows, the list can go on. (All interesting points of view; turn polarity.)

We have a built-in need to make each other wrong. This is not just simply a matter of having to be right most of the time. No, it is a built-in mechanism that says, "I'd rather be dead than be wrong." This is a major problem in our society today. How is that a problem? Because, folks, we don't take responsibility for our own shit. And as long as we can make someone else wrong, we don't have to.

And forget it if someone tries to help! Boy, talk about gotta-have-an-enemy! Wow, watch out. Yes, there is automatic voice that turns on when we receive help (it says destroy the helper) and the **mind** takes over and attempts to fulfill the command.

This make-wrong stuff of creating enemies where one did not exist before is of long duration. It goes along with the game of "me-against-them or, me-against-the-world" and so on, and continues the creation and existence of enemies of long duration and of the game itself. And the covert make-wrong is the most difficult to spot.

149

Run this quite easily and quickly by balancing Chakras and by finding and turning polarities on make-wrong situations.

- Pull and turn gotta-be-right-can't-be-wrong; sweep the entire body and look for incidents of have-to-be-right-can't-be-wrong;

- Find if-I'm-wrong-that-could-mean-death postulate.

- Find threat-to-life-if-wrong; turn polarity.

- Find can't-communicate-if-wrong; turn polarity throughout all time, all space, and all dimensions.

- Locate times of being helped—must-kill-or-make-wrong-the-helper—turn polarity.

- Just prior to the thought, creation, manifestation of decision to make-wrong, must-be-right, point of creation turn polarity, release and disconnect.

This may take some time to pull and turn as we are going to run into plenty of conclusions to make wrong; just stay with it and get all you can in one session. But please don't be discouraged if you don't get it all in one session, 'cause there is bound to be a lot of charge here.

End session with the light energy pulling from the head and scalp; balance the Chakras.

Run re-alignment, re-activation, re-creation, aging and

150

crown of manifestation.

Frequently Asked Questions and Answers

You mean even when we think we're taking responsibility for our actions and mistakes we may not be? I mean we must take responsibility for all of our actions.

We may be having people try to help and we twist what they say/do? Yes, this happens often. Yes, we come to a point where we realize we are responsible for everything.

Trap #2: Agreed-upon reality of mental illnesses

We Homo Sapiens can have, at times, a propensity to create and commiserate on similar states of mental beingness at the same time and in similar conditions including Hate, Fear Greed, and Depression (sadness) and so on.

Today we find many people in the apparently stuck conditions of depression and/or anxiety. Some are termed chronically depressed, others, bipolar. *Very interesting points of view turn polarity on each.* One thing they definitely have in common today is that these diagnosed conditions are great supporters of the pharmaceutical companies.

Now, I do not propose to say to anyone that has depressions or anxiety do not appear to *FEEL* real, or

151

they are not real. Hell, even "brook trout gets the blues." The thing is; many people give so much power and energy to the condition of depression that it reacts with more solidity of the unwanted condition. Or, some may resist it to a point of natural pull-in or habitual pull-and/or creation.

The suffering of depression does feel, in fact, very real and solid too many people. They sit in despondency, grief, loneliness, loss, separation and the feeling or sensation of heaviness, mass and concentrated force that holds one down and may contain the creation of continual crying.

The Medical community, AMA and pharmaceutical companies figure they have the answer (drug 'em!). And that very well may be the fix for some—not the best fix.

Included in this work is the avenue to relieve suffering on many levels, including the energy of depression, anger, grief, loss and many other unwanted emotions and sensations. And perhaps we'll eventually eliminate the need for drug therapy, just maybe!

Run this way:

- Start at the head; pull energy; pull from the feet, face hands and neck.

- Actually touch or hold these body parts and simply pull energy.

Folks, this stuff feels like a very hot vibration, and by now you should be attuned to what it feels like!

152

In the case of depression, ask the client to visualize the thing itself; to actually place the thoughts, creations, times, weight, mass, motion, color, smell, sensations and so on right in the palm of their hand—left or right hand or both hands, does not matter. Ask the client to describe the thing completely, what it looks like and what it feels like. Get all the specifics of the thing (depression) that you can; let them do all the talking. You do all the listening and all the remembering of what they say. And all the turning of polarity on every subject matter the client has brought up.

At the end of their telling, take each item and turn polarity for/with it.

This is rather interesting stuff; you need to get all the energy of the description of the thing itself completely and fully. This stuff will feel heavy and hot; you may even notice a turn-on within yourself when pulling. Not to worry, it won't last; as long as you keep blowing this stuff out through your crown Chakra and off to another dimension. In fact, you can run many emotions and unwanted conditions with this same process.

You will want to ask your client, "Where in the body do you hold this?" Get a response. Instruct the client to reach in and pull it out; hold it in the palm of your hand; and tell me what it looks like. Then remain quiet and allow the client to describe the thing completely. You can guide clients by asking more questions and leading them towards a complete description of the unwanted condition. Ask and let the client reply; what does it feel like? What does it look like and so on?

Turn polarity on all items the client brings up. This may take some doing as there is bound to be a lot of stuff to pull and turn. Ask for higher self-guidance to help get it all.

Trap: Mobius strip syndrome

Be sure to run the client's need to re-create the thing itself. Many people have the propensity to re-create the unwanted condition almost as fast as it clears. Why? Because 1) it gives the person an identity, 2) gives the person a game or something to do, 3) has become ingrained as cellar memory level dis-ease, 4) some just simply do not wish change or improvement in their world. It may be part of the Mobius strip syndrome[23], and you will have to get them off it. 6) Some people just really don't desire improvement. Hell, they just might actually have to do something if they were better, and we can't have that, now can we?

On all subjects brought up by the client, run same as turning polarity on all other subjects and origins.

Example: On the subject of depression (containing the thought and projection one must be depressed, as a means of healing karma, point of creation); turn polarity. Turn polarity on all thoughts, ideas considerations creations, implants, projections, judgments on: needs, wants-to-have depressions; turn polarity throughout all time, all space, and all dimensions; turn polarity, just prior to the thought prior to creation of depression turn polarity, release and disconnect.

When you see a shift in the environment, reality, condition, or appearance of your client then end the session.

[23] Mobius strip syndrome = a figure 8 on its side, running into infinity, never ending, always on the same path

Finish the session by sweeping the body and asking for or calling up re-alignment, re-activation, re-creation and re-newel.

Once again, folks, you may not get all of this in one session. There is bound to be plenty to handle from many lifetimes and incidents of depression, anxiety, multiple personalities and a whole host of AMA term dis-eases. Please just keep at it; this is the stuff that will change and improve your client's life and assist in leading towards an improved experience on this plane.

According to the Dalai Lama, when we relieve the suffering of a negative mind we can experience happiness and an enlightened experience here on planet Earth.

Frequently Asked Questions and Answers

This stuff has a temperature? I mean it's hot or cold?

Yes, hot or cold is correct.

We can help other people not to be depressed or mentally ill by our actions concerning them?

Only occasionally

Trap #3: Lifetime of memories, get rid of them!

This is as simple as it gets, folks. Go after all the cellular memory, mental memory and brain memory that you can, which creates suffering in/on one form or another. Remember this: "the mind is a wonderful thing to waste". Get rid of the mind completely, and you get

155

rid of suffering; that is what Christ was referring to as evil (the mind that is). Live in the here and now and let your work be done—with the exception of emanating love wherever you go.

The important point to keep in mind is that you are going to have to get people off the continuum to create, the need/want to re-create unwanted conditions and all forms of suffering. Re-creation works rather automatically and is, for the most part, people are not aware of this. And we must get the infinity of creation off the Mobius Strip of creation and the Double Mobius Strip and the trap of all time, all space, creation of the unwanted conditions to re-create themselves automatically. The Mobius Strip is the #8 symbol turned on its side, which stands for infinity and creates the continuum of the cycle of suffering. It acts just like a rat on running on a figure 8 and can't, or won't, get off. You must work to get your clients, and yourself, off the Mobius Strip in order to end, or at least decrease, the amount of suffering one endures in this life on the plane. You can and, in fact, must pull the 8 symbol itself.

Plus, if your client can't, or won't, let go of suffering, you are spinning your wheels and will forever. If you let them by trying to "fix" them or rid the conditions or the thing a person believes they want to get rid of, man that just isn't going to happen! In reality, we are only assisting clients in their work for clearing. You cannot do it entirely for them.

If the client does not require, desire, request and demand change, improvement, more fun and a lighter experience on this planet, nothing you do will be of any help. Sure, you will bring about temporary relief but permanent change- *not*!

The process to end the continuum of suffering and break down the Mobius Strip:

Start by pulling energy up the through the crown Chakra from the feet and the entire body.

Run your hands over the Chakras; manipulate the energy in order to bring balance to the Chakras.

Locate time, place, form and event of instillation on to Mobius Strip. You locate the 8 symbol same as all other items with this work: by intuition and by the way it feels (check the solar plexus.) Turn polarity on all incidents, times, masses and so on. Get the original time (point of creation of the thing itself: The Mobius strip); point of creation, turn polarity, throughout all time and in all space, all dimensions; turn polarity, release and disconnect.

Turn polarity as cellular memory; turn polarity.

Find the 8 symbol and pull it; pull all symbols connected to this charge, including crosses and stars.

Pull Mobius Strip as mental memory.

Locate; back up—double or hidden Mobius Strip. Run same as above.

Find point of creation of Mobius Strip as brain memory, point of creation; turn polarity, release and disconnect.

Turn polarity on the thought just prior to the point of creation to all suffering in mind, cellular memory, brain memory, and mental memory as in recordings and so on; turn polarity.

Get the self-determined postulate to suffer, the habit of suffering, the addiction to suffering, the willingness, unwillingness to give up suffering.

Go after all self-created, self-surrendering, self denial, agreed to, accepted, wanted, needed, required, requested, re-created ideas, conclusions, concepts, resisted, put up, put out, put in place in order to create suffering in the here and now, get heart's desire to suffer for self abasement; turn polarity on all the above throughout all time and all space and all dimensions.

Get the weight, mass, color, shape, and smell, depth and so on to all suffering throughout all time, in all spaces, on all dimensions point of creation. Turn polarity; release and disconnect from Mobius Strip.

Get all resistance to suffering; turn polarity on all.

Have the client say "I, _____, do hereby release all needs/wants to agreements for suffering; I recount, rescind, recall and reject all suffering on my body, aura and spirit, in the here and now on all dimensions." I break all contracts to stay connected to Mobius Strip and agreements and previously held thoughts, ideas and concepts to suffering. I release and let go of all suffering here and now. I agree to release myself from the Mobius Strip.

Have the client repeat several times per day for several days:

"All of life comes to me with ease and joy and glory as it does you..."

End session by running re-creation, re-activation, re-construction, healing, sadness, joy, and creating life forms and crown of Manifestation.

Run your hands over the body. Check for any and all missed masses and balance the Chakras.

"When all beings are free from suffering we shall live in peace."

White Buffalo Speaks

Frequently Asked Questions and Answers

You mean that suffering has weight, mass, color, shape, smell and death? I thought that suffering was a feeling. You make it sound like a thing.

It has elements of all the above it can definitely be felt and considered a thing.

Trap #4: Get free from Machines

Mechanisms, grids, wormholes, implants—sounds like some pretty Sci-Fi stuff, doesn't it? Not to worry. Remember, folks, this is all about energy and it all flows. The thing that some people have trouble recognizing is that we can control the flow and direction of energy and have power over the ultimate outcome of our lives.

For many it will do well to practice just moving energy from one object to another. Let's say, for instance, take

159

a cup, a pot, a saucer and move energy from one object to another, get it moving around and around in circular motion. If you are having trouble doing it, just imagine that you are moving it to start with. Soon you will get the **vibration** (feeling) of actually moving energy. For people in the workaday world who are having trouble being in and making things happen in their environment, this is a wonderful practice. Just move energy from one thing, person or place to another. Soon you will find that you are having an easier time doing your work and making a success of it.

Practice this every morning soon as you get up: Go outside; pull from the environment the energy that you require for your enhanced experience. It works better than a cup of coffee. That's right, pull in energy from the trees, the mountains, and a blade of grass, the rocks, the ocean, and a car, whatever. Say to the Universe: Fill me up. Provide all that I require, desire and request to bring about a full, joyful, gleeful experience. Put your hands out or up. Ask for all that you desire and feel the radiance of the thing itself, occurring in the here and now.

Pulling loving energy helps to vibrate your desires at the same time; i.e., hummmmmm, I would love a new car. Get a picture of the car and radiate or vibrate the thing in the here and now. Ask the Universe to supply all that you require to pull in the car to you're here-and-now reality. Release and allow the Universe to do the work and offer thanksgiving for its delivery in the here and now. Do you have trouble believing it? Well, fake it till you make it; works better than not trying at all.

Now on to the next subject, this is mechanisms, grids, and implants. It's all energy, right? We have been slammed, bombarded, electrocuted, shocked, starved, beaten, placed into, drugged, put in, barred from, cut off, scraped, shredded and torn apart. Not to mention brainwashed by contemporary federation corporate media (governments, advertising and the news).

Now, it's not all bleak and, no, I'm not accusing anyone of turning anyone into a victim.

We can get ourselves free from the grid (slammed into sort of a computerized field), we can disassemble mechanisms (machines that hold us in place), and create the ideas "to do the right thing, do what you are told, walk the line" and so on. "Well, I-can-only-do-what-I-can-do syndrome." We can, in fact, despite the locked gate of implants[24] (hidden, out of sight), open it up and free ourselves from the conditions agreed to in the contents of the implants themselves.

Contemporary implants come from television news and advertising, along with conditioning of hunger, overwork and fatigue. Other implants of today's negative processing can come from radio waves, electrical impulses, cell phones, microwaves, army training, shock therapy and drugs.

Many of the above-mentioned items can, or have been, placed in surgically implanted and/or put in by some means somewhere on the body, usually the head the nape of the neck. Don't get all bent out of shape; you can handle this as well—just pull it as energy.

The way to pull the above-mentioned items is to start at
[24]   Implants = forced, shocked, placed-in ideas and considerations, usually from a source of long ago. Often from evil sources, such as the Federation

the head, <u>hands on the body using only your fingertips,</u> pull energy from the crown Chakra, and pull from the base of the neck, the third eye, the hands and the feet.

Often, you can create and pull your clients' favorite color through these areas or just pull the color light blue throughout.

Ask for specific implants to come up; ask for electrical shock, and ask for other or earlier lifetime surgical procedures; find and spot implants that contain phrases, like "I can't" or "you just never know!" "I couldn't hurt a fly," "No, don't do that; you'll hurt yourself," "yeah, buts," "tried," "there is a reason for everything" and about a million other recordings people play over and over again. The more you get to know your client, the easier it will be to spot implants and mechanisms.

Run point of creation on all of the above.

Implants and mechanisms <u>removed</u> bring about marked improvement in your client's life, with increased freedom and allowance for individual responsibility. Once you remove implants you will see your client start to take off and fly.

This may require a little patience as you will find it necessary to run implants on a regular basis since there is a lot to do here. Plus, crap bombards us on a daily basis as well.

Pulling one from the grid, implants and mechanisms are easy work once you know how to spot them and know what you are you looking for; i.e., repeated phrases and language, which create a handicap or disability.

When pulling one off the Grid, look for thing-no-thing at the same time, as it may have been included within this trap. Thing/No-Thing fits well into, "I don't know". Ask someone, what's wrong? No-thing/this thing/I don't know. It's a trap of pretending not to know, or blocks one's ability to know and cuts communication—turn it.

End with re-creation, re-activation, re-alignment, and crown of mystery and manifestation.

Frequently Asked Questions and Answers

You mean we can get energy from things that don't have life?

Everything has life to some degree we are all made of the same stuff, only some life forms have choose to have more intelligence, when bugs no longer want to be bugs they will move up the chain.

So if I want something, like a new car, I just claim it?

I'm not really quite sure what a new car has to do with this? But, yes, just claim it.

Trap #5: The desire to die or destroy

It may seem unreasonable, but it seems some folk's just want to quit, let go, stop, die or destroy something once created. Why? No reason, it's an implant of sorts. It says, "I must succumb!" This is a rather strong postulate and has destroyed many lives, careers,

163

businesses, and civilizations.

Find the succumb postulate and turn it

Find the need-to-destroy-what-was-once-created postulate, held in the heart Chakra, and is usually hidden. Simply find the postulate and all back-up mechanisms, turn, and pull them to all points of creation.

Frequently Asked Questions and Answers

So we die or destroy something because we feel we're supposed to?

It's a trap and a lie, probably created by the federation and we just went into agreement with it. Yes, turn polarity on dying.

Chapter 26 – Other Areas to Work

The following is a list of items that you will want to search out and handle with you clients. You can work all items listed below with same procedures as described above. Just run your hands over the body and find what charge has connected to it. Once you do find it, just run it.

Also, you will after doing this work for a little while, you will come up with new, (fresh) discoveries that will resonate with your clients that need to be handled. Ask for higher self-guidance and go for it, just pull and turn whatever comes up. Remember this: if your client shows signs of worsening, that's OK too; it's just a stage of the work. Continue; be determined and all will work out just fine. When the client indicates or looks like there has been an improvement, end session and ask them to tell you what happened.

Go get 'em

Walk-ins to the original occupant, Galactic Mesh, Galactic Monster, Destroyer, back-up Destroyer, Thing-No-Thing, Shadow Self, Past Future Mysteries, Immune System, and False Immune System. Pull Ego; Back-up Ego, and all egos. Pull the Symbol of the Cross as being a self-created barrier to success and/or fulfillment in one's life. The symbol of the cross comes to us from ancient times (pre-Christ). It can have amazing beneficial qualities as well, but can also contain a trap, consideration of a stop, pull and turn the negative effect of the symbol of the cross in all cases.

Pull and turn all this, as above; continue

Pull Body-Soul Implants and The GE or Genetic Entity. Pull all Symbols of Historical Religious creations such as crosses, stars, staffs, light symbols and so on. Pull Wormholes, Worms and all Parasites. Turn Polarity onTunnels and release from Black Holes. Find, release; and turn Portals. Do Dimensional Doors; Dis-eases, Malfunctions, breaks, sprains, and times of unconsciousness. In-capsulated Cellular Memory on the spine, In-capsulated Memory of all head points in-capsulated on the spine. This is deep level work and when applied with artistry will change an aspirant's life completely.

Some of the above-mentioned items may sound a little far-out. They are all implants of long, long ago and need work. They <u>all</u> will show up on your client eventually, and are very much worth checking and working to remove. And, you already have all the data there is to process these items. Run all the above to points of creation, turn polarity, release and disconnect, as discussed throughout this book.

Frequently Asked Questions and Answers

Some of these things sound like science fiction, out of space stuff coming into our bodies or something.

Yes, it does, I know — but they are in fact real and need addressing.

If we pull things out and get rid of them, can we also mistakenly pull good things? How do we know the difference? If we think we've pulled out the wrong thing or things, what should we do?

166

Trust, Faith and just do the work, you will FEEL the difference and like I said before, people are not going to release what gives them pleasure, just doesn't work that way.

Chapter 27 – Clearing the Being

Let's see if we can just get this thing cleared up once and for all.

The mind that is.

Give the instruction and affirmation, "Mind, quiet."

Run mind-clearing and pull all blocks to a quiet mind. Ask client to repeat the phrase, "Mind, quiet." Pull all stops to a quiet mind.

When Man/Womankind can rise above the mind and come to the realization of our God/Goddess-hood, we will find there is no need for the mind. And, we can have perfect peace, even without the need for meditation, because there is nothing upon which to meditate. We are IT.

Yes, the body/brain does function in order to keep some GE[25] in the process of running things; we all know that, and that is not what I am referring to here. To what is it that I refer? Why, that little devil that doesn't know how to quiet down on its own! It thinks in terms of "everything equals everything else," and does not know how to differentiate thoughts or perceptions, it just thinks.

What I am suggesting is that we can realize our essential self, allow our knowingness, be conscious of

[25]   GE = Genetic entity, genes are believed to be responsible for the optimum running of the body, the genetic entity is an implanted reality based on opinion, not on truth or its power

ourselves in the here and now; be one with all sentient beings and all living things, and drop the concept and the need for thought and separation brought about by genetic theory. "All thought is good for is something to do" A great unnamed philosopher; "everything else that it creates is havoc". This is provable by observation; just look at people who think a lot—they're nuts.

The little devil mind just goes and goes and goes not unlike the *Energizer Bunny*. The only real and true creator is the person himself or herself—before now known as the "I". And the "I" does, in fact, know all and does not have to think about anything.

Yes, the mind runs into its own wanting-to-survive postulates, its own duality, oppositions, needs and wants, chains of reactions when threatened, and so on. The thing is, the person inside the one in charge, the "I", does not require a mind to operate on any plane. Why? Because the mind is useless; it does not function from knowingness; it functions from the viewpoint of thinkingness and nothing more. Thinkingness is a waste of vital energy and gets one nowhere! We know everything there is to know, right here, right now. The only good that comes from saying to oneself " I don't know" is to decrease one's ability to know.

Yes, the mind will come up with all kinds of tricks to aid in its own survival. After all, it does not want its own destruction. One will notice, particularly after giving instruction, "Mind, be quiet", that it, in fact, will/can become more active. The mind will/can turn on to a point of nearly driving one crazy. When your client has this sort of occurrence; have them simply say, "Hum… interesting point of view," turn polarity, and allow for the turning and return to mind quiet. All sorts of thoughts, emotions, sensations, considerations and so on will come on; hum... interesting that the mind, the brain, cellular memory can have this effect, interesting point of view, turn polarity; mind quiet. There is no effort required for the instruction, mind quiet, just tell it and allow it; yes, it takes some processing but in my experience, anything worthwhile does take a little persistence.

The process to gain control over the mind is to tell it to quiet down and go away.

And allow it to do so!

Be Mind Quiet.

Sweep the body for all mind functions. Find visualizations, masses, weights, smells, visions of others, thoughts, ideas, oppositions, considerations, thinking-ness, mock-ups, postulates, creations, opinions, counter-creations, emotions, projections, loss of power, judgments, solidities, barriers, blocks, walls, dark rooms or places in relation to mind, and pull and turn polarity on each. Run to point of creation, turn polarity, release and disconnect on each of the above. Run to original point of creation and all points throughout all time all space in/on all dimensions turn polarity, thought just prior to original point of creation, turn polarity—release and disconnect.

If you notice the mind becoming more active and noisy, it is actually stimulated into activity and is just a little fired up. Why? It wants to survive. It wants control and does not know the difference between good control and bad control. When you notice the brain/mind activity in progress, don't panic. Rather tell the client or give instructions *go into complete allowance*, as much possible and allow the noise the activity, the havoc. Yes, simply experience the thing (mind) quietly and completely. *Hum, interesting point of view that the mind could be this active.* Almost enough to drive one crazy, interesting point of view, point of creation, turn polarity, throughout all time all space all dimensions, turn polarity—release and disconnect. As the noise turns on heavier or quiets down, repeat, "Interesting point of view," turn polarity. The idea here is not to fight against or resist the mind activity at all, what we resist tends to persist.

This stuff works, folks. I'm not writing this information down to see my words on paper- I am sharing information with you that can very possibly change yours and your client's life to a point of amazingly beautiful and seemingly incredible out come. Apply it, process yourself and your clients to a quiet state, allow the mind to quiet, and your experience on this plane will become more a thing of joy rather than confusion, fear, anger and separation. I invite us to step into Love, Peace and Joy with Glory, Prosperity and Oneness; living in perfect health and retaining these bodies for a very long duration of time.

Mind quiet.

Give the instructions to the client to instruct the mind to quiet and quietly allow it to do so.

When I refer to solidities of the Mind, i.e. considerations, thoughts, and so on, of course I am referring to things being solid, stuck, hard mass that helps create and hold in place the mess (BOXES) we are in and we are in solidly. The idea of this work is to become less solid, less fixed, and freer to experience pleasure and growth on this plane. When we are free to create, paint, write and focus on the real purpose of the "I", everyone will be the beneficiary of our creations, or at least everyone that can appreciate what and who we are.

By the way, this isn't just this lifetime process; the results can last for many lifetimes or incarnations to come.

The Mind, Quiet instruction can be done on a regular basis and should be requirement of the client to do on their own. This process may seem unending, as there is a lot to deal with on this subject. Be patient and work it; you'll be glad you did.

End with sweeping the body to align the Chakras; call up and activate re-creation, re-alignment, re-activation and renewal.

She found herself experiencing perfect love, peace and joy with a perfectly quiet mind.

Men and Women can live on planet Earth in perfect peace and joy, living in complete harmony and glory with God and Nature—believe it—be quiet and experience it.

One last additional technical note: Be sure to instruct you clients to drink plenty of water while receiving sessions and to take as much salt and sugar as they feel necessary for their bodies.

Frequently Asked Questions and Answers

You make it sound like the mind is a bad thing, but don't people need their minds in order to know things?

No, people know things. The mind only knows confusion. "I am" knows all

If we get rid of our minds, aren't we leaving ourselves open to be controlled by someone else? * Not at all, we are gaining control over ourselves.

How about a break for some fun?

If Only Dogs Taught Us ...

When loved ones come home, always run to greet them

Never pass up the opportunity to go for a joy ride

Know the experiences of fresh air and the wind in your face
to be pure ecstasy

Let others know when they've invaded your territory

Take naps and stretch before rising

Run, romp, and play daily

Thrive on attention and let people touch you

Avoid biting when a simple growl will do

On warm days, stop to lie on your back on the grass

On hot days, drink lots of water and lie under a shady tree

When you're happy, dance around and wag your entire

body

No matter how often you're scolded, don't buy into the guilt thing and pout... run right back and make friends

Delight in the simple joy of a long walk

Eat with gusto and enthusiasm. Stop when you've had enough

Be loyal

If you Love him/her come when you're called and needed

Never pretend to be something you're not.

If what you want lies buried, dig until you find it.

When someone is having a bad day, be silent, sit close by and nuzzle him or her gently.

Be as easy to experience as you want others to be.

Back to work

There are vital elements to one's ability to rise above what heretofore believed impossible in the field of spiritual awaking. Today's discoveries may seem a little esoteric and even weird from the outset.

The mysteries to the unlocking the being from entrapment and finding the unfoldment of the soul are well known to only a chosen few mystic's, zealots, and universal practitioners. That was once the case. Now all practitioners who look closely will find all the answers they have sought after for millions of years.

Power Touch leads one to the unfoldment and final realizations one seeks.

Chapter 28 – Welcome to Power Touch

The first thing you should have noticed and should understand is the principle, point of creation turn polarity, release and disconnect. Add draw back your power; live in the here and now.

* Definition; all incidents, all that occurs all items of interest we are looking for have a point of creation, and all can be turned if they are undesirable, and released.

The practitioner's job is to find (incidents) them, spot the charge connected to them and turn polarity until all charge or attention on the subject dissipates and is clear. Once this happens, the client becomes free to make sound decisions in the here and now, to guide their future. Find the charge and relieve it with your hands. The instructions are repeated several times within the chapters of The Gift of Touch, as above, and this new work: Power Touch.

Frequently Asked Questions and Answers

When you speak of point of creation, are you sort of talking about going back into time to where something began?

Yes, exactly, now you got it!

Chapter 29 – What is Power Touch?

Power Touch is utilizing vital energy of the Gods in cooperation with all sentient beings to bring about positive change, a final and permanent healing. To help people come to a place in their lives living in perfect love peace harmony and joy with all other beings and come to the final realization—the unfoldment of the soul.

Power touch is taking your (facilitator) innate power and abilities to disperse energy, create miraculous change and bring into existence a healing for your brother/sister Homo sapiens.

When one realizes his/her connection with spirit and gives into the power to heal through touch, one can certainly assist in creating change in ones-fellow life's partners worldwide, as well as one's own life and that of others in search of love peace and joy.

Power Touch will create the changes you are after as a practitioner for your clients and as aspirants seeking knowledge, truth and God, that so many are doing in multitudes of modalities today. Is it possible to live a complete life full of joy, prosperity, and happiness; in perfect health and well-being for a very, very long time? Yes, it is, and Power Touch holds the promises we have been seeking for thousands of years.

Even from the earliest days of Vedanta, Hinduism, and Buddhism, up through to Christianity, Sufism, Shamanism, Science of Mind, Access, and Scientology man has been in search of a way to heal his fellow man and help relieve his/her suffering.

Today, with love and science combined, what has heretofore been seen through the eyes of philosophy and religion has taken a new form of science mixed with love to bring about a desired result. A healing, healing through the simple manipulation of energy flows in and around the body of one in need of a "HEALING."

Frequently Asked Questions and Answers

So, power touch will let us change things for our clients so that they can lead a complete life full of good things? Will their lives stay this way? Will they need to be treated? Should they have the energy manipulated on a regular basis?

Unfortunately, it looks as though there always might be something to process. The more awake we become the more we have to confront, deal with and release. But, it is also a good thing. The more we release and let go of the brighter and lighter we are.

Are you saying that some of the things taught in religion are now being shown to be true through science and love working together to be true?

Science and religion have come together, yes.

Definition: To heal. To bring a person to spiritual wholeness. To create well-being.

The student of Power Touch will come to recognize their personal power combined with love for their fellow man to restore wellness, wholeness and well-being in/with/for the seeker of truth and well-being. Practitioners who become interested in the work should be prepared to approach this work with one thing in mind-the desired outcome! The results we are after come through science and love. Love for your client, all humanity, plants, animals and the scientific approach of this work.

Frequently Asked Questions and Answers

So power touch is more than just a manipulation? You actually have to feel a love for your client?

Yes, but please recall that started in part one of the Gift of Touch.

What if someone schedules an appointment with you; shows up; and you just don't find them lovable? I mean, what if the person is really a disagreeable person with a chip on their shoulder and a "prove it" attitude towards the help you desire to give?

It may be so that we do not resonate. We have a choice — for the client to seek work elsewhere or to stick with it and assist the client.

Again, what is energy healing?

Energy Healing is the ability to change conditions, strictly through the application of manipulating energy for the good of all.

Power Touch is an extension of my earlier works on the subjects of massage and energy healing. My first book on the subject written in 1974 Major Breakthrough in Massage Technology covered very basic considerations of the mechanics of energy flows that are still relevant here today. In my second book the first part of this book now, The Gift of Touch 2001 covered the subjects of energy healing. The main idea that energy can become locked or blocked, then dispersed or released and thus creating even flows are still applied today.

Science has proven that energy can be blocked, locked, or turned off, and can move in a rather uncontrolled hectic or dispersed manner. In this we took a look at many subjects relative to relieving suffering and bringing about a more desirable state for human beings, strictly through the manipulation of energy and the removal of various blocks. Through Power Touch, I shall deliver new and relative subjects in need of address to further our understanding and ability to help our clients and ourselves live happier and more fulfilling lives by relieving blocks and suffering.

What I hope to illustrate to "healers"-practitioners/facilitators is that when energy if flowing, naturally, evenly and gently aspirants will experience well-being, wholeness and vital life energy flowing through and around their bodies. This is spirit healing on its deepest level. I hope to encourage you to open yourself up to the power to heal through Power Touch.

Through the application of simply asking energy in the environment of the client's body and aura to shift, and in connection and direction of Spirit and the assistance of great ones who have come before, we will work to relieve suffering from aspirants that have given into considerations that has lead to their suffering. For it is ideas, postulates, concepts, decisions, agreements, considerations, resistances and so on that has lead to our entrapment, unawareness and sufferings origins, and there-by free us all from suffering and assist in our allowing a more pleasurable experience here and now, here on planet Earth and beyond. It is with the application of asking energies to shift and turn, that

Homo- sapiens will find their true self and their freedom.

Freedom to operate with new found abilities, free from others energies, free from blocks and locks that tend to hold one down, oppressed and suppressed from being who they truly are, joyous, loving beings able to create on many levels or dynamics and being of loving service to all other sentient beings. Free to live an optimal life full of joy.

Frequently Asked Questions and Answers

You make it sound so much as if energy is a physical thing that one can take hold of and manipulate, yet energy is a force of some kind, isn't it?

Yes, it is both.

Are you saying that practitioners working with power touch are working together with other beings that have lived before and are still alive on some other level or something?

We can indeed connect with powers outside of ourselves and procure additional help.

Do you mean that people give into certain things that cause their suffering?

Yes, we go into agreement or resist the things we don't want; or we vibrate them in one way or another.

The Problem or Challenge

Has been going into agreement or resisting others energies that got us into to trouble we are in, in the first place. While it is true there are no victims, we have managed to get ourselves trapped into beliefs, through agreements or resistances to ideas, considerations, postulates and decisions of others. Or the resistance to them! The aspirant of personal freedom and the unfoldment of the soul will do well to learn very quickly and completely, Emm, *very interesting, point of creation, turn polarity, turn polarity throughout all time and all space and all dimension, turn polarity release and disconnect*-a subject we have covered in length in earlier chapters.

*Notice unwanteds: Just as an exercise: Emm interesting point of view turn polarity, release and disconnect. Do this on a daily basis, every time you notice ideas or energies coming at you, that are not your own and you choose **not to own them.***

The subjects we will cover here all have to do with controlling energy and disconnecting from blocks, locks and barriers on a somewhat more esoteric level.

The aspirants (clients) challenge is-once released is to NOT re-create that which is gone. A challenge to be sure; one must learn the principles of Mind-Be- Quiet, a subject coved in The Gift of Touch above, and we shall cover again here.

Through the loving art of meditation mind quiet one can break through the walls of bondage, of illness and dis-

183

ease, free from sadness and able to achieve ones hopes and dreams. Yes, strictly though the application of manipulating and channeling energy flows one can live a completely healthy, happy, satisfied life, and be one with the Creator and all other sentient beings.

Go into mind quiet, much healing occurs there.

Frequently Asked Questions and Answers

Do you mean that we cause our own problems by accepting certain things or rejecting certain things?

Yes!

You said in one part to get rid of the mind, now you're saying something about going into it. I know that I'm missing something, would you explain please?

Go into it completely and fully, experience exactly what is there and allow yourself to let it go. If one resists an IT, it will just get bigger and more solid. Once it is gone, one feels lighter, brighter, and gains ability to work on this plane, until ready to ascend.

Chapter 30 – Who Am I?

Who am I and what am I doing here? This question has plagued humanity since the beginning of time. Would you be surprised to know that not many people have had the opportunity to find the answer to this question? Even through many, many life times of asking have past. Why? The answer lies hidden, veiled by many life times of confusion, dark spots and being off tract or off purpose and being deeply invalidated, and implanted.

I Am

To start with, one must be willing to know! The block of unwillingness to know needs to be turned and pulled. Why would one resist knowing? What are the consequences of knowing? Mystery of Knowing Revealed! Knowing requires one to wear their responsibility hat, not such an easy experience for some people. Once we know who we are and what we are doing here, one becomes responsible for their life and finds they must take action to make their life happen the way they desire.

What is the result of taking responsibility? A glorious life form full of creation, free from doubt, fear and the unknown, free from considerations that help hold one in place or down trodden and free to create the life one chooses. The only way people can complain about government and other entities suppressing them, is if they don't know who we truly are and what purpose we have in being here.

There has never been a time in history that man/woman has not ask this question. Who am I? What is my purpose? What is my work (reason) for being here?

Some may have a built in pretend I don't know, some may dramatize I can't know, fearing harm if they did know and others may simply mistakenly choose not to know.

But millions of people today do want to know. People desire to live the life of their dreams; people want to live happily, healthy, prosperous lives. If one denies this, they are lying to themselves. The desire to know is so strong that countless millions of people spend their entire lives in books hunting the answer to an appearance of a mystery that lays beep in the center of their own hearts.

Who am I and Why? The answer will surprise you but has always been there, even since the beginning of time.

Having and knowing one's vital purpose in life is as basic to life as clean air and water, and more so. Knowing who we are and what we are will aid us in knowing why we are and the why is always supreme. Discovery of who I am I and why come through the process of turning polarity on not knowing. Can't know, shouldn't know, and too dangerous to know. Take each item, turn polarity on it, and allow one's self to come into knowing. It's really quite simple and will require only a few hours of processing. If one chooses not to know anymore, that is their choice. * turn polarity to not knowing as with all processes listed in above chapters. This is essential processing for both client and practitioner

Frequently Asked Questions and Answers

So, if we existed before and exist now, is who we were then a part of who we are now?

Yes, most definitely. We carry whom we are over into each incarnation until cleared.

Do you mean that it's not completely a clean slate starting over but rather a growing continuation?

It can be either depending on one's state of awareness.

Nature of knowing

There is a Native American principle that says, "When one knows who they are, and their path, they will walk it their entire life." And all one needs to do is get out of one's own way and ask. The answer will come. In native practices, one goes out into nature, quiets one self and asks the primal question, who am I and allow the answer to come. (Please see *Open Spaces: My Life and Times with Leonard J. Mountain Chief*) This could take a day, a week or a month and in some cases years.

I ask you do the same thing; quiet yourself and ask, and the answer will come.
"Come into scared ceremony, and come out transformed!" Leonard J. Mountain Chief

This is a primal question, if you or your client already knows who they are and don't have any charge on the subject, do not process it. When you do notice charge on the subject that needs running, you may bring up heavy emotional charge with your client. Stay with it run it until it cools and your client comes to new realization of who they are. To get this might require more than one session. Put on your determination hat and get it. This is so powerful you "will wake the dead." I guarantee it.

Frequently Asked Questions and Answers

So what is a life? Is it being one person or is it your entire existence?

It is all there is. Yes, it is one's entire existence, and you cannot ever destroy life.

Can a practitioner and their client form a sacred ceremony?

Yes, people can enter scared ceremony at any time; come into sacred ceremony in silence and reverence and come out transformed. Being out in Nature is the best way this is accomplished.

Processing Not Knowing

Have client lay face up on massage table, shoes off. Practitioner ask client to lie on their back quietly and breathe. Instruct client to ask who am I and repeat the question throughout the session.

Start by bringing balance

Start by balancing the Chakras. Sweep your hands over the client's body from head to toe, reminding the client to breathe and relax. Continue the question "who am I," throughout the session.

Process

Run your hands over the client's body; call up times of not knowing who they are, turn polarity, and feel for the charge you are after using your hands. Continue running your hands over client's body. Call up:

- Can't Know

- Refuse to Know

- Unwilling to Know

- Won't Know

- I can't Know

- Dangerous to Know

Frequently Asked Questions and Answers

You say call up, ok. Suppose they come forward, do they talk to you? I mean, are these actual entities? What do you do with them?

Yes, sometimes they are entities. Shake hands with them and then process them. Call up the means to activate, call near and to process it.

Remove all barriers to knowing

Turn polarity on whatever charge you find

Spot hidden knowing

Back up can't know

Hidden mysteries to knowing

Millions of years of I don't know who I am

Comes up as I don't know

Turn polarity on what comes up to not knowing who one is, what they are doing here and what they are

Find times of pain and unconsciousness in relation to knowing turn polarity

Ask client to continue to ask who they are

Who am I?

Continue to sweep the body and find where the charge is; pull the charge turn polarity, throughout all time all space all dimensions, release and disconnect

Ask the client to continue to breathe, relax, and ask, "Who am I?"

Soon the client will run out of reasons to not know and come to understanding

Once you have pulled and released all of the charge on not knowing, the client will come to know themselves and their vital purpose.

Now set a new direction

I, _____ *state your name*; speak for my client_____ *state their name.*

Here and now, break all contracts to not knowing. I, now, in this time place-form continuum, agree that I do know who I am and now take full responsibility for my life, all actions, and all results. **I Am**

Rebalance chakras

End session

Have your client write out on a piece of paper in a concise statement who they are and what their purpose is. Have them hang this up where they can read it on a daily basis.

There are polarities in everything, situation and being-ness in all universes. Turning polarity requires a practitioner to turn hot from cold, positive from negative, good from bad, white from black, light from dark and so on. When we turn enough polarity on a subject the charge, connection, and attention cool off. You have restored a spiritual being's innate attention and the person is whole.

When we experience well-being and light-ness, a healing has occurred.

191

Frequently Asked Questions and Answers

You speak about hidden things. Can you know things about the client that they don't want known or is there a way that they can maintain their privacy and only reveal what they feel in necessary or what they want to reveal?

By looking deeply and by feelings one can see everything

The Procedure

The practitioner uses their hands to sweep the body of their clients to find blockages, remove them, turn polarity on the charge, have it release and help the client to allow the charge to release. Have them state new postulates for a new behavior in life, which will lead them toward healing, wholeness, knowing who they are, and what their path, or direction in life is. The practitioner moves his/her hands inches off the body to assist in finding dark, hot or vibrating change from the clients body and aura.
We also work hands on; particularly the feet hands head and spine, heart, third eye and tummy; the client always remain clothed.

Frequently Asked Questions and Answers

The client is in control then? That is, the client has to release the charge?

We are working together, and client never gives up

control.

Chapter 31 –Take a Walk

When we find ourselves very confused, depressed, anxious, and not knowing where we are, it is time for a walk.

The Process is simple, go outside and take a walk. This is causative walking. It is a cognitive way to ground oneself, get located here on planet Earth, relax, find centering, and obtain healing.

Whether bothered by our life, our environment, jobs, spouse, family or circumstance, we need to take a time out and walk. **This is best done in Nature.**

One does not have to be in a low emotional state to take a walk. Take a walk daily, and as a meditation instead of an achievement.

The process is to go outside, go to a park or out in the woods and walk.
Breathe & Walk! Notice the environment, touch objects in the environment, and find out where one is instead of where one is not.
Just walk, breathe and look.

The flowing is from my book *Open Spaces: My Life and Times with Leonard J. Mountain Chief*, enjoy...

Come into sacred ceremony, come out transformed!

The Ways of Nature

Delivered to me, through Leonard, about the things of nature and the spirit world we call home:

"Look here my son; do you see the way the fire burns in a circular motion? As in a wheel of medicine? So it is with all things in Nature, even you and I. We are here and then we are not. We are there only for a little while, and then we are elsewhere, forever moving in the four directions of the fire circle."

"There is no other way. Everything is in one place for only a moment in time. It cannot stand still. That is what made The People nomads for many thousands of years. We are one with the fire, the sun, the earth, the water, and the air. They are in constant motion. We are that. There is no other way."

"We are like birds in flight, moving in one direction or another with only one thing in mind—to survive. There is no other way. It is our Nature."

"It is in that mountain. Watch and listen to her very carefully. Sit quietly. Do not speak of her. Observe her. Hear her. It is all Nature. Sing the Nature song and dance with her. She is a wonderful partner. It is her nature."

"Hear the song of the flute and you hear my truth. Walk the way of the Red Path and you will see. Walk the way of the bear and you will see there is no difference, it is in nature, and there is no other way."

"When the drum song plays and we dance, we imitate the animal world and in our dance of the animal world our nature is revealed. There is no other way."

"When the woman of your dreams hears your song of

195

the flute, she will come to you, there is no other way. It is her nature. Only the natural world can take man and woman by the hand and show them the way to walk."

"When you arrive at the mountaintop, you do not arrive there by riches, you arrive there by heart. There is no other way. It is Nature."

"When your brother calls out to you to come to be by his side, you must go. There is no other way. It is his nature to request you to be there and yours to respond. You must go. There is no other way."

"The natural world holds all the answers. It is in the sweat lodge, the dance, drum, and song. It is in the trees and the running water. It is our nature to hear the words, to hear the message of love or war, of fleeing or standing still. There is no other way."

"Man and woman can walk this earth together, but without Nature there is no way to hear or see the Creator and He may not speak to them at all if not through Nature. There is no other way."

"My son, everywhere you go there is Nature. Look all around you as you walk. As you speak from the heart, notice Nature. There is no other way. Walk barefoot on the earth every day."

"Hear the elk cry at night. It is his nature. Observe the coyote dance, hear the song he sings to his brothers. There is no other way."

"When you consume the herb, know from where it came. It came the only way it could, through Nature. There is no other way."

"Listen as you have before. It is in the wind. It is in the sun, moon, stars, and planet Earth. It is in the very soil you love so much. Nature is crying out to you, 'Hear me, hear me!' There is no other way."

"Nature holds all lessons for you every day. Will you play? Will you stand still? Will you listen? Is there any other way?"

"Look to the East, and the lessons of new beginnings. Turn to the West, as the sun sets and brings a new rest. Face up to the North and find a time to be still. Gaze down upon the South and allow the healing that you require. The time has come to stay and experience. It is nature. There is no other way."

"It is all here for your asking, without the slightest struggle. It's all here for you now, and it is free. It is Nature.

"Give thanks and praises to the Creator. It is in the circle of Nature and it is your path to look after her. There is no other way."

Leonard often spoke of Nature and the importance of listening, to hear her speak. He taught me to become silent and conscious of Mother Earth's needs and to protect and love her. "What you give her, she will give back to you a thousand times," Leonard said. "It is in her nature; there is no other way."

On one occasion, I said to Leonard, "So much oil, gold, silver, and oil is up in those mountains. Why doesn't the tribe harvest some?"

"Because we like it right where it is, Jay," he replied. "It is in our nature."

"Be in Nature," he pleaded. "Be with her daily. There is no other way."

Come into sacred ceremony. Be quiet and listen; there is no other way.
Go now and daily, take a walk, there is much healing to be experienced.

Frequently Asked Questions and Answers

All of this is beautiful and poetic but is it something that we as people can actually do? Can we enter into One-ness with nature, and what does that mean?

To be it and be One in it.

Chapter 32 - Cellular Memory Processing

Being free to create the life one chooses

The body is like a computer that holds tremendous amounts of data, in Cellular Memory. Once we start deleting this negative unnecessary information in the form of blockages within your body & mind, one feels healthier and lighter – physically, mentally and emotionally stronger. This is a way to freedom.

For billions of years, beings have been trapped by beliefs and implants held in by cellular memory force, in or around their bodies. Now, in this millennium, we are finding new ways of becoming free and living happier, more productive and prosperous lives. Living as we truly are, glorious creators, living in bliss with other grand beings.

One of the traps essential to keeping people down and entrapped is the Cellular Memory Implant and freeing ourselves of this implant can have extremely valuable results. It is the job of the healing practitioner/facilitator to help his/her clients through the barriers that hold people down and keep them trapped, towing the line for the *federation.

* The Federation is a historical society (organization) of long standing, or long time tract, an evil empire, they refer to themselves as royalty. Their mission is power and control. Evidence of their power is experienced through domination, high cost of living, high or outrageous tax system, unjust laws that only protect the wealthy, prison systems, world banking, global mega-

business, oil and industrialized war machine are their tools used for controlling others.

We are all creators, teachers, writers, artists, leaders, and healers. The federation does not desire that we know this, and becoming free of cellular memory implant will lead one to your own unfoldment of the soul, thereby allowing beingness of who you truly are – a free creative soul, living in harmony with self, the environment, all other peoples everywhere, and all living things and creating in Love, Peace, and Joy, free from federation control, thereby changing the vibrations here in this plane and ensuring our survival as Homo sapiens.

Cellular Memory Processing will open the gate to the spiritual attainment people have been searching for; The amount of blocked energy stored as life's charged incidents is rather dramatic, and the opportunity to unlock this charge to be made available as positive energy flow will dramatically change a human being's life for the better.

There has been a code discovered and the way to open the flood gates to allow this charge to be released and the code is 12346789201, using this code for the process will open the gate and allow the charge to be pivoted or be tuned. It is an implant.

What is cellular memory? It is blockages, stops, barriers, incidents, thoughts, ideas, considerations, concepts, projections, contracts, pain, discomfort, agreements, resistances, and beliefs held on, in or near the body on a cellular level. Times of consciousness or unconsciousness held in the body, mind, brain, spinal cord, and aura, held in as trapped energy that saps one's energy and depletes ones attention and ability to operate in a here and now environment.

Trapped by cellular memory implants!

Processing is worked to relieve all cellular memory and release a being from the effect of cellular memory implants, thereby freeing one to operate at optimal levels on planet Earth, in all areas of one's life.

Frequently Asked Questions and Answers

Cellular memory? Code? This sounds like computer stuff. Would you explain more on this please?

Yes, we have been implanted with several codes and implants. Cellular memory processing will help to break the code and return one to his/her innate self, removing the computerized trap one can tend to live in.

Examples

1) Lower back pain caused by injury, held in place by the body cells to create suffering based on memory principle. 2) Chronic headaches held in place by restimulation of cellular memory implant 3) thoughts, ideas, considerations, opinions that are in fact detrimental to ones survival are held in place by cellular memory. 4) The body holds incidents, the brain holds incidents, specifically the spine, hands, feet head, mind and aura are all lock boxes for cellular memory incidents being locked and hidden from aspirants view. 5) An incident is a time of trauma/drama and agreement, it can or may hold unconsciousness and always holds degrees of charge and attention units. 6)

Releasing cellular memory blocked energy will open one's ability to be here now, experience nowness and create in a present time/space form, which equates to a happier, more stable, creative individual, living in present time, free to expand ones area of influence and responsibility. And be in their bliss.

Cellular memory was introduced several billion years ago by beings referred to as doctors as an implant to further entrapment beings, by the federation. Beings were also trapped to go into agreement with its power and effect at the time of original implementation a code was inserted to unlock the chain.

The code must be verbalized each time a practitioner works to unlock the effects of cellular implants and the code is 12346789201.

Working to unlock cellular memory processing will not be effective without first using the code. In the procedures below you will find out how you use this code and find cellular memory implants and turn the effect of them and freeing your client and/or yourself from its effect.

Human beings dramatize the effect of cellular memory implant by showing signs of insanity, erratic behavior, rapidly changing thought patterns, moodiness, lack of stability in livingness, unable to concentrate or focus attention, in chronic pain, mis-emotional, severe disabilities, dis-eases and chronic low level emotional states; such as fear, sadness, anger, grief and fixation on death. Applying the process that follows with clients may take more than one period of time for session. One may find a multitude of incidents and each need to be turned to original point of creation.

The practitioner/facilitator will find original point of creation and agreement by the client to be the effect of cellular memory. When that is done to its completion this process is done. If one does find additional charge in the area continue to run the process until clean and no charge remains on the subject.

Frequently Asked Questions and Answers

But if cellular memory was produced billions of years ago, even if reincarnation is real, we have different bodies now so wouldn't that mean new cells? So how would these new cells have what is in the old ones?

Cellular memory travels along with one.

Practitioner, working with client

Client lies comfortably on their backs on massage table, with shoes off; their body position will need to be changed from time to time to allow access to the spine.

Begin procedure by simply asking client to breathe, relax and allow the procedure to be run. Ask clients permission to run procedure and ask for their agreement for cellular memory to be released. Ask client to take a few deep breaths and relax. Place you hands on client's body in several places and allow client to experience your touch. Following instruction to client is, normal breathing and relax.

Then began processing by running your hands over the client's body, about four inches above the client's body and balance the chakras. Once energy is flowing smoothly and client appears relaxed start cellular memory processing.

Process command as follows:

Cellular Memory Implant Open 12346789201

On a cellular memory level (pain) or whatever the subject is, held in the body as cellular memory, turn polarity, turn polarity throughout all time, all dimensions, all spaces, all places, forms, events, turn polarity, at time of creation turn, release and disconnect. Continue, just prior to the agreement to accept cellular memory implant, turn the thought, turn polarity throughout all time, all, space, all dimensions, turn polarity, release and disconnect. Important, call up cellular memory for the subject that you are working, by asking, i.e. concerning headaches on a cellular memory level.

Close your eyes and call up 12346789201 ask cellular memory implant to open up to your access and you will feel the gate open.

Begin be sweeping the clients body, or your own in cases of solo processing[26], and looking for cellular memory implants, speak aloud whatever you find and ask it to turn. I.e. Times of unconsciousness and pain on any subject you are running on the client, **sample,** time of injury to the lower back held in place by cellular memory implant, feel the charge and ask it to turn. Point of creation turn polarity, throughout all time, all

[26]   Solo Processing = working on one's own body to relieve suffering

spaces, all places, and all dimensions, turn polarity **release and disconnect**, repeat until the charge dissipates or cools down.

Important note: when you ask that the energy of the subject to turn polarity release and disconnect ask the client allow it to disconnect and allow the energy to flow out through their own crown chakra **without** the need to re-manufacture or re-create that which you just dissolved. That is you just turned for and with your client. Ask the client to allow the energy to release, allow it to be gone, and so it is.

Release and disconnect, allow it to be gone! Continue this command during the duration of the processes.

Then move to touching client's body, with your hands or fingers, work the feet, hands, head and spine.

Frequently Asked Questions and Answers

So the client does it with you. Is the client aware of all that is happening?

Always stay in communication with the client. Yes, they know what is happening.

Call up and ask for cellular memory implants of:

- Pain

- Unconsciousness

- Agreement to be the effect of_____

- Ask for times of agreement of cellular memory connected to whatever subject you are after I.e.

- Beliefs

- False beliefs

- Belief's from others

- Grief

- Losses

- Addictions

- Effects of emotion

- Times of injury

- The appearances of lack

- Trauma

- Assault

- Rape

- Murdered

- Betrayed

Note: client <u>does not</u> need to reply verbally

Find Projections connected to suffering:

- Judgments

- Agreements

- Contracts

- Ideas

- Projections made by client him/her self

- Thoughts

- Problems

- Challenges

- Considerations

- Opinions held on all of the above

Handle each, and all are held in cellular memory in the hands, feet neck head, spine and Aura, be sure to clear aura thoroughly. Run all of these experiences as being seen by client to self and others to self and others to others, this picks up all four *flows.

* All four flows, experienced by self, self to others, others to others, others to self

Frequently Asked Questions and Answers

Client to self, others to self, and others to others. That only sounds like there "three flows" not four. Would you explain please?

Yes, and done to client makes four

Note; asking for the clients agreement is important, we all made agreements to be the effect of cellular memory implants, we agreed to it under stress. And asking for and finding times of agreement will help to relieve this charge. None of us are victims we all went into agreement with this and other implants, finding agreements helps to lift the effect of implants and take responsibility for our actions and to become conscious of our decisions to base future decisions on, and allow

The unfoldment of the soul and reach our full potential as spiritual and human beings.

Each time you find charge on a subject you are working run POCTP, point of creation turn polarity. All subjects a client comes into session with can be run with cellular memory processing. This stuff is powerful folks and please do not discount the effectiveness of running this process. The outcome will be nothing short of miraculous.

In session work the feet and hands completely leave no part of the feet, hands, head neck and spine untouched as it appears that is where the these implants have been placed and hold the most charge.

Use enough pressure on the body as the client needs to feel these areas being touched and they will also feel the release.

Frequently Asked Questions and Answers

209

You speak of this as being powerful. Is there anything you can do to make or allow this to get out of hand so that it is an endangerment to anyone in any way?

Reply

There is no danger in personal power, as long as we don't abuse it

Find the It

Find what **it** is for each client, find out what **they** are being the effect of in/on the body and aura. Call it up on cellular memory level (whatever **it** is for the client) call **it** up on all parts of the body as mentioned above. I.e. on a cellular memory level oranges make me sick, find where that is held in the body on cellular memory level ****POCTP it**.

Each client will come in with an **it**, could be pain, could be emotion, dis-ease. Whatever their original **it** is needs to be run till complete, then dig a little deeper and find the REAL **it**. There will always be the earliest **it** and the original creation of the **it**. Find the core **it** and you will change your client's life forever. Run the **it** with POCTP on each (**it**) item on wherever you find **it** held in the body. Find original **it,** find point of creation held in cellular memory and turn it, and you will have a vastly improved client.

Be sure to remember to turn the clients body on either side or their stomachs to work both sides so that the spine can be easily accessed and work each vertebrae on the spine. Ask for and call up the subjects you are looking for in relation to clients request and complaints about their bodies and or lives. Run each item to POCTP on a cellular memory level (that means to process each thing to completion, until cools down completely). It is cellular memory we are after here and the **it** connected.

Very important

Be sure to run the list of items mentioned above and work to completion. Run what the **it** the client comes in with and the **it** on each item until complete. If a subject has no charge, it has no charge, find the ones that do and "turn" them.

As with other processes, work this with 25* PCOTP on each subject on cellular memory to completion. If client continues to suffer, run agreement to suffer process and un- willingness to heal POCTP on all subjects.

25* PCPTP, short for point of creation, turn polarity

When client FEELS complete, work to balance the chakras and call up re-organization, re-creation, re-activation, re-newel and ask the client to break the contract to suffer, from the effects of cellular memory. Ask them to set a new postulate for today's livingness based on a glorious life, free from being the effect of cellular memory, free to create, free to be responsible for self and others, free from the effect of cellular memory on the body mind and spirit. So it is, end off.

Procedure in 1, 2, 3 magic!

Ask client if they would like to run this procedure

If they agree,

Have client take off their shoes and lay face up on massage table, use pillows to support head and under knees

Ask client to take three deep breathes and relax

Touch client's body with your hands and ask them to notice feeling your hands. Move energy.

Run hands over client's body 3– 4- inches above ask them to continue breathing and relax, balance the chakras

Call up 12346789201 ask cellular memory implant to open up to your access and you will feel the gate open

Sweep your hands over client's body and find places where these implants are held on a cellular level

POCTP each item you find. Clear them release and disconnect. Ask client to allow release and disconnection from cellular memory. Find every subject available

Move to touching the client's body, hands, feet, head base of neck and spine

Run the list above and run each item until complete (no Charge)

Whatever reason the client came in with ask for the item on a cellular memory level, run it until complete and then get the **it**. The **it** will be core for their issues, run **it** until complete, release and disconnect.

After all items feel cool and complete run your hands over clients body again and see if anything had been missed- be careful here to not over run, but don't leave it undone.

When client is complete, run your hands over their body once more, balancing chakras and call up reorganization, reactivation, recreation, renewal.

Ask client to allow 4-6 weeks to notice changes in their lives and to report back to you often, re-run process until complete.

This process will change your clients life forever and can be the balm, please let me know how it goes.

26*The Federation an evil empire of elitists founded over six billion years ago, these beings are embodied today as politicians government workers, politicians, business-people, attorneys, police and military and controlled by the very wealthy, known as the illuminati in contemporary earth terms *POCTP is short for point of creation turn polarity.

* All four flows; done to self, self done to others, others done to others, witnessed others to others and felt the effect.

26* The Federation, evil empire set up by those who consider themselves royalty to entrap all other being as slaves, IE; high gas and food prices and indentured servitude through high taxes. Set up on a rock planet six billion years ago.

Frequently Asked Questions and Answers

What if this takes longer than you expected and the client's time runs out? Can you put this on "hold" for t he next appointment?

There is always work that can be done, stop at a comfortable stopping point for both yourself and your client. Or, continue as long as there client has attention on the subject and not fatigued.

Chapter 33 – Create the Life You Have Always Dreamt

This is a training course designed by Jay North to help you live the life of your dreams. When it comes to creating a bigger, more abundant life have you ever thought, "Some people have all the luck"? It's easy to think of good fortune as predetermined. Either you've got it or you don't. *But in actuality, karma is only a small part of the equation. Attracting good fortune, or getting lucky, is actually a fairly straightforward process. When you recognize your talents, open to a bigger vision and use your intuition to help you make the right decisions at the right times. There's no stopping you! Your BIG vision is already becoming your reality. So it is…*

"Create the life you want" has been a hot subject in the last hundred years or so and approached by millions of seekers.

All you need to get there is to know where you are going

As an exercise: Meditate daily on nothing!
Allow it to be done and experience it in the here and now.

When life gets too confusing and you just can't seem to get a grip on it, here is the formula: First, stop everything!
Occasionally all one needs to do is just stop, look around, and find out where one is. Then, make a plan

for where it is you think or believe it is you want to be, do, and have.

Stopping does two things. One, it gives you the opportunity to relax and just listen and find out who you are and not who you are pretending to be. Often it's when we are at our quietest state that answers tend to come easily, without force, worry, or concentration. Two, stopping allows creativity to flow. When we are so busy thinking, fretting, and praying for a change, we are just too busy to allow creative freedom to flow. Just stop, breathe, relax, and listen.

Frequently Asked Questions and Answers

Do you mean we should sort of lay claim to the way we want things to be, and live as if they already are that way?

Yes, absolutely.

Sometimes starting begins with stopping, even if just for a moment Find a rock

Once several years ago, while I was living on the Blackfeet Indian Reservation in northwest Montana under the tutelage of Leonard J. Mountain Chief, I had many worries and concerns going on in my life. Everything just seemed so over-whelming. Leonard took notice of my despondency and suggested an old Indian practice: when the people find there is just so much going on in their minds that they feel lost and confused, they go find a rock.

The practice is simple. Find a rock and focus all of your attention on the rock for as along a period as you can. If you find your mind overly active or just can't seem to quiet down, "allow the experience" and return to focusing on the rock. Staying focused for as long as you are comfortable is the way it works best, <u>as long as you are comfortable</u>. It could take minutes, hours, days, or weeks, and perhaps in some cases even years, to come out knowing. One always knows when one FEELS complete. "Allow the experience," means to get as comfortable as possible and simply experience it. Experience exactly what is going on in

---

As an exercise: See the picture, events, forms, and success as already done, on a daily basis, for one week, or one month, or for one year. Visualize daily.

---

the moment and allow yourself the experience. It eases concentration on the rock. Trust me on this one, please. Just allow and concentrate.

When we're able to stop, get located, or find out where we really are, we can then proceed to a process of our own choosing; or with the assistance of a trained facilitator in life planning, we can undertake our life's (re) organization.

Frequently Asked Questions and Answers

Does this simply mean to stare at the rock; or to examine it and learn all we can about it?

Yes, just look at it.

Write it out!

In a perfect world, it starts with visualization and belief. Write it out.
Start here: in a perfect world I would have, do, and be. Creating a plan for our life does happen to require a bit of work—real life actions. There are several components to consider. Whether creating a plan for work, money, life, or love, the essentials—having a specific purpose, goals, and a map—remain the same. The components are actually many. Access them in a uniform order. They could and should be flowed to the "T"[27].

What you visualize in your life and <u>believe</u>, you will achieve. In a perfect world, what would you want to achieve?

Where is it you want to be, what do you want to be (i.e., "Being-ness" or identity), what do you want to have, and what do you plan to <u>do</u> to get it? In a perfect world, consider what you would have, do, or be. Visualize it, believe it, and you will achieve it.

It is interesting to note that within the definitions of the words "have," "do," and "be," the common denominator is "create." What are you willing to create to possess, create yourself to be, and what product or service in life do you choose to create to be a benefit to others? Creation is the key ingredient, no doubt. This means taking responsibility for our lives, something not easy to experience for some Homo sapiens. So, more exactly, in a perfect world, what are you willing to create?

---

[27] "T" refers to Triumph. It means living, doing the heretofore thought impossible.

> *As an exercise: Write yourself a memo and paste it in a place that reminds you on a daily basis of determination, persistence, and consistency; and add your personal confidence to stay on track.*

Frequently Asked Questions and Answers

Do you mean if we want something to exist in our lives, all we have to do is picture it as being there and it will be?
Hold on to the vision, vibrate it, and it is done.

If you have a good picture (visualization) in your mind of exactly where you want to be and exactly what you're true desires are, and you believe in them, you are half way home. All you need to get there is to know where you are going. But, get it out of your mind and on paper. You are going to need a map, a drawing, and a written plan that you plan to stick to for whatever duration of time you have allowed yourself to reach your goals, hopes, and dreams. Creation in the mind alone tends to be a confusing picture. On paper, it becomes more solid, less confusing, and real. What do you desire, require, or request?

The subjects are vast; the choices are many. But the basic principles remain the same and constant whether it is a successful career, home, and family; saving the planet from nuclear destruction; or running for public office. That is as close to an absolute as one can find! After you become completely quiet and come out to look, ask, "What do I desire, require, and request in my life? Deep in the center of my heart, what do I really need and want? What is the greatest good for the greatest number?" Service could be a key factor here so take a close look.

Not to be a joker, but what if you picture yourself as running for public office and winning; and someone else does the same thing; and you both believe? What happens?

Where there is construction, there is always destruction. It is part of the planet's game. No two shall occupy the same space at the same time. Although remember now, a "win-win" can also be found in every situation.

Start by looking and being honest with yourself

Creating the life we choose to have, and life organization planning, require one to be totally honest with oneself, determined and persistent in achieving the THINGS we believe are important in our lives (e.g., abundance, peace in our homes and country, a successful career, marriage and family, clean air, pure water, or whatever it is you truly want). It requires courage to look and to <u>act</u>. It requires confidence in one's choices; specialized knowledge, ability, or training to reach specific targets and goals; and the courage and confidence to bring them into the here and now.

> *As an exercise: I allow what I desire, require, and request into my life in the here and now.*

Start with stopping. Stop everything you are doing and/or thinking you should be doing, even for just a very short period. You will come to a realization, I promise. Then you can begin the journey of visualization and creating the life you want, but only after you have become quiet and know.

Here is a valuable tool: Once you know what it is you truly want, write a plan based on what you really, really want. Write it in the <u>past tense</u>. Write every paragraph as though whatever it is you want has already come into being or has already happened, and then give thanks to the Universe for supplying it.

Gratitude goes a long way with regard to getting what we want.

The way this works is that, you postulate[28] yourself, or it, into existence. By writing in the past tense, you are deciding that the thing has already taken shape and form in the here and now and that on the basis of metaphysical principles, it has no other choice than to respond in kind. Acknowledgement is the key deciding factor in the creation of the thing itself, hence gratitude.

Another important factor for aspirants to keep in mind is time line and dates. Assign an exact date (also called a target) as to when you expect things to happen. Never leave a decision or a conclusion just dangling out in the Universe waiting to happen.

While we're at it, whatever your thing is, and if you

---

[28]   Postulate refers to a decision or a conclusion based on past data to help guide one's future or "nowness."

desire support from the Universe and the people in it: (1) never stop communicating about it; and (2) use this law: Outflow Equals Inflow. The Universe will always reply with an inflow of comparable magnitude to whatever you outflow. Recall the Buddhist principle of cause and effect. It's a principle that one could live by ones entire life. The degree to which one generates outflow is the degree to which one will receive inflow, and your personal power in life depends on your willingness and ability to generate outflow. Outflow love; get love in return. Outflow money; get money in return.

It's your life. *"All you need to get there is to know where you're going."*
- Jay North 1977

As an exercise: Life is in me today. I never regret yesterday and I make my own tomorrow.

Look at it this way: this is your life. Why not make it the one you want? Go out into nature; find a rock. Be quiet and listen. It will come. Know (visualize) what you want. Make a plan, but be flexible.

As an exercise: I never disparage my own strength or power.

Formula Expanded

Life planning

In a perfect world I would have, do, and be. Write it out completely as a road map or a painting. Plan by what you want or that which you want to produce:

- Who are you really?
- What are you?
- Where are you?
- What do you really want?
- What are your hopes, dreams, goals and purposes?
-

If you intend to sell a product or service, what are the:

What are the goals and purposes?

- Plans?
- Projects?
- Programs to make this happen?
- What is (are) the real job(s) that must be done to succeed?
- What policy shall you set to make sure this happens?
- What are the targets?
- What are the statistics?
- What does the ideal scene look like?
- What is the valuable, viable final product?

Visualize daily. Meditate. Be quiet and breathe.

The business world—here it is dry in "the real world!" This is for creating a business plan according to academia:

- What is the product or service?
- What are the goal(s)?
- What are your principals' backgrounds? WHO ARE THEY?
- How much financing do you require? Energy (MONEY)!
- What will you do with the money?
- How long will it take to pay it back?
- What's in it for investors/backers?
- What is the scope of the endeavor?
- Who are your customers?
- What is the product exactly?
- What are the income projections?
- How will the product be marketed?
- Who is your audience?
- What is your marketing plan?
- How will you let your customers know who and where you are?
- Location, location, location!
- What is your advertising plan and costs?
- Who is the competition? What makes you better?
- Are your services and products better than your competitors'? Write it out.
- Who are the board members or partners of the business and their backgrounds?
- Plans for establishment. When will you be in business?
- Targets with dates.
- Conditional targets. What do you need to do in order to be set up?
- Bookkeeping and accounting.
- Savings.
- Taxes.

- License.
- Insurance.
- Benefits.
- Plans for expansion.
- Vacations.

Knowing what we really want is the key to creating miracles in our lives.

Write down your postulates. Write what you expect to have achieved by the end of the day, each day, and each year. Decide and write what you would create by the end of the week. Expect the outcome to occur just the way you see it. Remember to write it as though it already happened. Do not overlook the creation of timelines and dates for goals you want to accomplish. They are vitally important.

As an example:

At the end of 2020 I re-created my business, my personal life, and myself. I am healthy, happy, and have prosperity. My income grew by $100,000 in this PAST year. My new mate loves me completely as I do him/her. And I have discovered a way to have a stronger and healthier body.

Postulates, conclusions or decisions

On a daily, weekly, or monthly basis, decide what it is you want to achieve. See it as already done. Assign it a timeline and definite date for final accomplishment. Never leave a postulate dangling in outer space waiting, or it shall continue to do just that—wait. Keep a journal and work from an appointment book.

In the cases of achieving hopes, dreams, and big important goals, see it, believe it, have faith in it, and know it. But more importantly, emote it. FEEL the emotion of the thing having already happened! What does it FEEL like to earn a million dollars, earn an important award? It FEELS fantastic, great, wonderful, exciting beyond words. Except now, your challenge is to find the words, then create the emotion as though the thing has already taken place here and now—get it, emote it. Positive emotion not only can, but also will earn you what you want in the here and now. It is a physical universal law that what we truly want and feel, we get. The Universe does not know how to operate differently. Similarly, if one expects to lose, one will.

Check your purposes. Does what you want align with your personal goals and purposes; or is it just something you fancy, like a new Mercedes-Benz, not that having one is bad mind you, but do you really want one? Does it align with your personal purposes?

Here's a daily exercise for the rest of your life: Decide what you want, check your purposes, set a timeline, and decide that it has already happened in the here and now. Acknowledge the thing done, and give thanks and praises to yourself and higher power for accomplishing the thing that you most want. Always pat yourself on the back and reward yourself. Continue to postulate. Move up in desires, if you so choose. Aspirations and goals are your own, and you must see yourself expanding in consciousness as you continue to grow and find the ultimate postulate—the unfoldment of your soul.

Live a life of expectancy, not waiting but accepting every wonderful thing you have ever wanted to come.

Make it a fun and lighthearted experience and even try to enjoy the bumps.

Here are your steps, as easy as 1, 2, 3:

- Go find a rock and be quiet.
- Ask and ye shall find.
- Who am I?
- Where am I?
- What do I want?
- What are my goals in relation to this?
- What are my purposes?
- What plans do I need to make to achieve this?
- What are the conditional targets?
- What projects lay ahead of me?
- What are my own postulates in relation to the goal and purpose?
- With whom do I need to communicate on this?
- What does the program look like?
- What decisions or conclusions do I need to make?
- How can I target getting things accomplished and sticking to them?
- How will I know things are moving along well toward achieving what I really want, or how can I set statistics?
- What is the ideal scene connected to getting what I want? What does the picture look like? Paint it!
- What purpose does it serve for others?
- And finally, what is the viable final product for?

Visualize daily what you want. Draw a picture, make a map, and see it in the here and now.

Breathe, relax…and smile.

The power of will power

What is really important? What are the goals, purposes, or achievements you desire? And what is it you want to achieve?

Once you have made a decision on these points, it's going to require your personal (innate, natural) power, or the power of your will, to accomplish whatever you're setting out to bring about in your life.

Willpower is the single most important factor in achieving greatness in any area of one's life.

Achievement requires: (1) visualization and seeing the thing as being done in the here and now; (2) focus, concentration, and follow through; (3) trust—open yourself up to trust that what you want is good, and just trust the Universe to support your efforts in the actualization of the thing(s) you want; and (4) WILLPOWER.

Imagine the power you need to transcend fear, worry, and inertia coming down through your crown Chakra and flowing out into the world to add the power, strength, and fortitude you require to see the thing to its completion. Inflow power, outflow power, and see the power of what you want as already done. Visualize it, believe it, keep it, have faith and belief in it as done, remain confident in your work and goals, and never, ever give up.
It takes courage, faith, and strength to achieve what we want, but our dreams are singly the most important

THINGS in our lives. There is nothing else. Use willpower and focus your energy. This can, and, with patient practice, will work miracles.

Finally, allow success into your own universe.

Frequently Asked Questions and Answers

Is there any special significance to the measurement of three feet above your head?

It can be any distance one is comfortable with.

The Power of visualization

Whenever two or more are gathered in common cause and can see clearly the destination they wish to arrive at, and can see the ride getting there and the reward, they can be in harmony, agreement, and focus; they shall create miracles. Visualize fully and completely what it is you want to have, do, or be. See it as already done and allow the success that you desire to be here and now.

Determination, persistence, consistency

When we set out to achieve what we believe we really want, and there is nothing else as important, it does at times require personal strength to stay on one's path, which requires determination, persistence, and consistency. This means the willingness to choose a path, create a product, and the power of singly focusing our attention to getting what we want. There are two tests for all beings to take: (1) create something out of nothing; and (2) never give up (not easy for the lighthearted). Once you find you have put in one's own personal ethics to achieve that which we perceive is important and the accomplishment of the goal, there is nothing more heroic. Nothing.

Here is a helpful practice: take up fly-fishing, golf, target shooting, archery, darts, or poker.

Learn to see the field. Opening yourself up to anything in the field is possible through targeting. While there may be only one bull's-eye, there are several areas or targets that one can hit. As in the games mentioned above, there are main or primary targets, secondary targets, and conditional targets; off-the-board shots or attempts that have little or no effect on the game; and there is winning. Using targeting as a gradual process, and accomplishing targets as one moves up in rank or into higher conditions, prepares one for more winning.

Winning at any particular game can at times be a gradual process, and using exact targeting assists one in the accomplishment of lesser goals or targets. Start with small targets, experience a win, then pat yourself on the back for achieving it, and set a new one.

Set priorities in targeting, and "star rate" them by importance (what really needs to be done). Acknowledge yourself when you hit a target; then upgrade and set a tougher target and hit it. Eventually you will find after a short period of setting and hitting various targets, you will be winning at the game you set out to achieve in the first place.

Used in the scale above, targeting fits into plans, projects, and programs and helps define your to do list. It helps take the mystery out of actions needed to accomplish in winning the game one has set out to play. When you hit a win, congratulate yourself and move on to the next one. When you fall short of hitting the target, say whoops and start again. It takes determination, persistence, and desire. Keep swinging, keep your eye on the ball, and learn to see the whole field.

Frequently Asked Questions and Answers

Do you mean like someone, sometimes uses a point of aim in archery that isn't the bull's-eye but will help us to hit the bull's-eye? For instance, if your arrows are hitting about eight inches to the right of the bull's-eye when you aim at the bull's-eye, you choose a point of aim eight inches to the left of the bull's-eye in order to hit the bull's-eye. Is this the same thing?

It's a very interesting question. Eventually you are going to hit the bull's-eye; just don't stop shooting.

Allowance and attitude

The single most common challenge people have is allowing themselves to achieve the thing they believe they want the most. This includes success in business, home, relationships, love, the unfoldment of one's own soul, and all deep desires. All one really needs to do is get out of one's own way and allow themselves to experience that which they truly want.

Allowance and attitude could be the biggest hurdle you will face in achieving the success you desire. One may have the courage to go after their dreams, they may have the belief and faith in what they are doing, they have applied *Determination, Persistence,* and

231

Consistency, postulated clearly, have confidence in their hopes and dreams coming into being, and have visualized the outcome even before it has occurred. The only challenge left is to allow and keep a great positive attitude about one's actions. In many cases there is going to be the requirement of processing to assist in removing barriers to allowance.

Process any and all areas of the above to remove blocks and barriers

I break all contracts, agreements, projections, and conclusions that bind me to self-sabotage, and I now allow myself to experience a grand and glorious life full of Prosperity, Abundance, Love, Peace, and Joy. I live in prosperity, I contribute a valuable service to planet Earth and humanity, and I prosper greatly for my actions. I have done little or no harm, and I now allow complete success into my life.

Write the above statement out and place it in view where you can see it and read it aloud on a daily basis. If one finds that allowance and attitude are major barriers or challenges, one can process this easily.

There is nothing senior to one's personal goals. There is nothing else as important. Your goals, hopes, and dreams are your own. Never give up and never say never.

Note to the reader: Some solo (processing one's self) processing may come up that needs to be addressed. This is easily accomplished. Just run POCTP (point of creation, turn polarity) whenever you notice resistance. I wish you the very best success in all areas of your life. I wish you the very best journey, and along the way, in the words of Leonard J. Mountain Chief, "Never stop smiling." Make the journey fun because "if it's not fun, I'm not going."

For individuals that have a product or service they wish to market on a substantial basis, I would highly recommend reading my book *Grow Yourself Rich.* Although it is written to or directed to an audience of primarily Organic Farmers, it is a wealth of marketing data I have applied over the past 30 years to market a wide variety of products and services. Please order your own copy from either website www.OneGlobePress.com or just call me and I will arrange getting a copy to you.

Please see new website for Jay's Books www.OneGlobePress.com.

I see myself as perfectly healthy, strong and vibrant. It is done.
I see myself in perfect health and vitality. It is done.
I am healthy. So it is.
I am living in my full potential and I am.
I am living my heart's dream and my path.
It is done.

Chapter 34 - Vibrate, Emanate the Life You Want

Following is a Special Message to Healing Practitioners From Leonard J. Mountain Chief, in agreement with White Buffalo Speaks,
Delivered by Jay North

> *What if humans discovered they were responsible for everything that happened to them? (Was Hurricane Katrina man-made? Was HIV?)*
> *Could we have a world without disasters, without war, without famine, and without dis-eases? Are there such things as cures? You bet there are! Do governments throughout the world or huge pharmaceutical companies want you (us) to know this? Hell no!*
> *Could we possibly postulate ourselves into a utopian existence?*
> *What would life be like without AIDS, cancer, heart dis-ease, starvation, street drugs, and crime? What would life be like without ignorance, murder, rape, and hate, jealously, greed, and power over those considered weak?*
> *What if we could live in comfort, love, peace, prosperity, and joy simply by adjusting our standard of living?*
> *Could we as a race of Homo sapiens actually find a way to raise the education standards throughout the world so each individual sentient being could have a chance for a decent income and the comfort of a safe home, clean water, productive, organic foods and enjoy their existence rather than toil in the mud for a grain of rice? Yes, it is very possible and doable. And you and I are here to create this, with love for each individual on this planet. It is our job.*

Governments won't do it. They would rather see people die than to be of true service, unless, of course, they find a way to line their pockets. (Whoops, sorry. No blaming here today, my dear, I promise.)

The more awake you have become, the more responsibility you must take

Can we find a way to be loving, sharing, caring, and giving far beyond what we may currently believe are our capabilities? Can we agree to be of service and expect a fair exchange from the Universe or God Mother for our deeds? Yes, we can and we must!

Can we be gracious to all people everywhere and say to them, "You are my brother, you are my sister, my father, and we are one"? We have been separated by fear, jealousy, anger, and greed for far too long. We come from the same place, you and me. We are one with the Creator and in HIM we shall find Love, Peace, and Joy and share it freely.

Now, granted some entities do not want us to know this or do anything of the sort. Some entities are pleased with war and destruction. Their very lives and pocket books depend on it or so they think. But what if...just what if...we could change our vibrations enough to allow, finally, One-ness and true unity? Could we come together in harmony, provide for one another, and wish one another Love, Peace, and Joy? Yes, most certainly we can. And we must.

The course this planet is on is not a very pretty one. We are facing our own extinction based on <u>our own</u>

postulates and decisions, or ones we have gone into agreement with long ago.

Can we, in fact, pivot our choices and set a new course? Yes, we must far long into the future, not just merely to survive, but prosper far beyond our current realities of prosperity.

We can actually reverse counterproductive postulates; de-stimulate their effect upon us; and set ourselves on a new course towards freedom and individual responsibility for the survival of humanity. This is essential and timing is critical.

As one of my very favorite teachers, Leonard J. Mountain Chief always loves to say, "There is nothing else." And, in truth, there is nothing else more important. This may take a little work, but so what. What else do we have to do...wash the SUV tonight?

In a perfect world, can we have, do, and be Love, Peace, and Joy equally for everyone, everywhere? Absolutely and we must!

Visualize this. About three to four inches just above your head is a light source of loving, soft blue color. In it is the radiance of the Godhead HER self, golden, beautiful, soft in nature, nurturing, loving and protective and ever powerful—full of love for everyone regardless of human considerations of who they are or what they may have done. Just visualize the light please.

Good. Now allow yourself the experience of this radiant light coming into your realm, into your being (body and aura), and allow yourself to become it.

Great! Now gently radiate this Love, Peace, and Joy out to the world and allow every living thing to feel its presence.

Very nice! Now have every sentient being in this field (planet Earth) feel loved and protected. Allow them to experience exactly who they are—grand and glorious creatures here—to experience a grand life just like you and me. And so it is.

We can change the vibrations on planet Earth. We can take the responsibility to ensure we have a place to play as does each and every loving mother, father, sister, and brother on the planet, regardless of age, race, creed, color, education, or current standards of living. War, greed, hate, crime—we are about to change all of that strictly and completely by changing frequency and vibrating. Let us, you and me, agree to hold hands in perfect harmony, right now, right here in this place. There is nothing else more important.

Vibrate Love, Peace, and Joy. Go ahead. Send it out. Allow each and every soul to experience its radiance, its joy, its love and peace. Use your power, flow Love, Peace, and Joy outward and simply allow everyone else to FEEL it. Flow it, don't force it.

Right now in this place

In this time, place, form, and continuum, we have a choice. We can go on, or we can accept the principles of Armageddon. The doomsayers want to be right. Groups on both sides of the cross think there is a better place in heaven. WRONG!

This is the place. This is our opportunity for freedom,

enlightenment, and unfoldment. This is the place of the soul's opportunity for freedom. Choose! This is not a war. There is no enemy. There is, however, choice; and there is emanation. This is the place for our children to play. There is no other like it!

Choose. Emanate. Flow Love, Peace, and Joy; and we will run together on a beach one day or climb to the highest mountain and look into each other's eyes and say, "Love, Peace, and Joy, we are here and so it is."

It has become of immense importance to change the harmonics on planet Earth before nuclear madmen end this time-place-form continuum. Peacefully dismantle nuclear power everywhere. Now is the time to vibrate Love, Peace, and Joy. Please join me.

> *Great Spirit In the Highest, Allow my mistakes and guide me the power to change the words an energy I outflow into and onto the world and out to the Universe. You have told us that your work is, all things together, for good to those who love you, to those who are the called, <u>according to your purpose</u>. I know you, I love you, and I am secure in your love. I know that your promises are true ones. I am, therefore, I am well, and I am, that I am. It is done… In deep gratitude, Amen*

Frequently Asked Questions and Answers

Does all of this require cooperation from everyone in

238

order to change the world for the better?   * Yes! But, it starts with you.

Emanate the world you want

Enjoy another story from my book *Open Spaces: My Life and Times with Leonard J. Mountain Chief*

This is important in the creation of our future.

There was to be a gathering, a Powwow of sorts, at the round lodge in Heart Butte. It was a time for dance and speeches from the elders of the Blackfeet Nations, and the only non-Natives to attend were married into the tribe or adopted. Leonard was to be one of the key speakers, and his subject on this day was family.

Pamela (my late wife) and I set up a booth for "Project Bluebird" at the event and gave a small presentation on our goals and projects for the organization. We knew about the event several weeks before it would occur, so we had plenty of time to create our booth. It was an honor to be invited and our intention was to make Leonard proud to have us there.

Pammy, as everyone used to call her, was also deeply in love with Leonard and had huge respect for him. She was very happy about my connection with him and always allowed me the time and space to be with him whenever he called for a one-on-one visit. She never felt left out, nor complained that I spent so much time with him.

One day in 1993, Pammy said, "Someday you will write about your time with Leonard and people will come to know him and love him just as you do, Jay." She was right.

Now, one thing I think I might as well point out is that everything on the "Res" is done in Native time, which means nothing gets started on time, at least not according to White man's concept of "on time." Pammy and I were very eager to get our booth set up, so when folks started to arrive they could come over for a visit and a short presentation to help them understand what we were up to. We packed our truck the night before and left the house at four a.m. so we could get to the lodge by six a.m. and set up. Thing was, nobody else got there till around ten. Some didn't arrive till noon. Scheduled to start at nine a.m., the event didn't really get going till around four or five that afternoon.

People wandered in around two p.m. and three p.m., and they were talking and eating the food put out, including my favorite, Indian fry bread. After a while, the drum songs started, and many of The People pulled chairs around in a circle to watch the dancing that started to take place. Leonard came over to me and asked that I join him in the circle and dance a while. I cried I was so happy to be asked, and joined in the dance that went on for several hours. Leonard remarked, "Gets you high, doesn't it? Who needs drugs? This is all one needs to get high and out of the body."

I laughed and replied, "Yes, Leonard. We do not need drugs. Our tribe is not a peyote tribe. It does not grow naturally in the area and we never use any substance for our visions."

The drumming and dancing went on for hours. We did not stop for water or food. We just danced, meditated, and prayed. After the dance was over there was a short giveaway, where grandmothers expecting new babies from their daughters gave away gifts in prayer for the child's good health and long life. There were gifts for the ill, the poor, and people in need on the "Res."

Then the chief of the tribe stood up and said, "It is time for us to speak." The elders stood up one at a time to name their subject and to speak on it. Some spoke about tribal politics, some about the water, others about the harvesting of timber, and so on. There were tribal leaders from all four separate regions of the tribe—two from Montana and two from Canada—where many of The People had fled during the last war with the Whites, in 1894, when the wars ended and The People settled. Then Leonard rose to his feet to speak.

"My brothers and sisters, we are one family," he shouted. "It is family that ties us and nothing is more important than this. We are one family and whatever disagreements we have ever had must end today, as we recognize that we are one family with our white brothers and sisters, and with dark-skinned people of all Nations."

Leonard asked that we quiet our minds and allow this family into our experience. The People looked upon him with wonder, some with enthusiasm in anticipation of what he was about to say.

"Quiet now," he said. "Quiet your mind. Breathe deeply. Relax and breathe. Close your eyes. Breathe. We are one family. Breathe and allow your mind to become quiet...whatever noise you hear, whatever pictures appear...and allow them simply to pass through you

241

and on their way. Breathe. Relax your brain, relax your head, and relax your facial muscles. Let the tension in your neck and shoulders melt away. Relax and breathe. Relax your entire body. Breathe into your chest and abdomen. Relax. Let your hands fall to your sides. Just drift and breathe. Relax your ankles and toes, and breathe."

"Now, notice a small purple dot right in the middle of your forehead, between your eyes. Feel this dot as warm, loving, and comforting. Breathe and be with this purple dot," said Leonard.

"Breathe. Now expand the purple dot all over your face and head and allow it to radiate down your chest and back and cover your body, back and front, tip to toe. Feel the warmth and love of this dot all over your body. Do not worry if it becomes arousing. Allow yourself to experience the joy. Now push the dot outward to include the energy around your body, and then out to your neighbors sitting right next to you.

"Allow your family to feel the compassion and love and happiness created by the purple dot. Let the purple dot fill the room and have every person in the room feel the gift of the purple dot.

"Now push the purple dot out to cover the entire tribal Nation and allow all of our people to notice its radiance. Continue to breathe. Relax and push the purple dot out over the Nation of the Americas and allow all tribes, all people, to feel the warmth and peace.

Love for the human family

"Expand your dot to include all people everywhere and allow them to be your loving family. Allow all people to feel your love for one family and all creatures. Allow the tobacco plant to feel your loving, healing energy and ask in prayer that all do the same.

"Breathe. Relax. Breathe love, breath peace, breathe love, breathe joy, and breathe love for one family everywhere. Allow the purple dot to become one purple dot, shared in harmony, love, compassion, and joy by all beings everywhere in all universes, and let it be. Be silent and breathe."

After a few minutes, Leonard said, "And now, as you come back into this room, in this time and place and begin to open your eyes, know that there is no war, there is no separation. Know we are one family. From this day on, we exclude no one from the way," said Leonard.

In the year 1994, the four Nations of the Blackfeet that had been separate for nearly one hundred years came together in peace and to reform as one Nation.

Training routes to emanation

It all starts with imagination and then follows through with emanation. Imagine the flow you desire your mate to feel. Imagine the result you desire in your home, business, and in the world. Create it and emanate it. Outflow through your third eye, root, and/or heart chakra.

Sit quietly. Face your friend or partner. Gently look into their eyes and allow yourself to be "there" comfortably for a period. Imagine, create, and outflow Love to your partner. Flow it outward from you third eye chakra.

Practice emanating love, peace, joy, acceptance, allowance, and harmony. Practice each of these creations individually and to their completion.

Now, expand the thought vibrations to include others in your family, friends, and circle of connections. Expand your loving influence out into the world and allow every sentient being to experience its radiant glow of Love, Peace, and Joy. Include all plants, animals, and all living things.

Emanation in practice is as easy as 1, 2, 3 . . .

Imagine, create, emanate, and outflow. This is our only assurance of survival on planet Earth. When you speak, speak only from the heart and emanate Love, Peace, and Joy. Vibrate, emanate, the life you want.

Chapter 35 – Attitude and Healing

Hazrat Inayat Khan, in one of a series of books Sufi Teachings, states how important attitude is and how it affects every part of our lives. Khan defines attitude as the most important element in our consciousness that brings about healing to our bodies, minds, and souls.

Have a great attitude and take fewer pills

Many other prominent writers, philosophers, and higher thinkers such as Deepak Chopra, L. Ron Hubbard, Earnest Holmes, and the Dalai Lama have each said in their own way that our attitudes in life and our thinking create our realities. What we think, what we say, and what we do defines not only our lives but our general health as well. Change your words and change your life, or more adequately put, "Change your story, change your life!"

You may take "laughter therapy" with any other medicine or treatment you choose, and it may be taken with or without food, as desired. There are no side effects. You may take joy and laughter along with any other treatments and therapies. Just be careful not to split a gut!

As long as we continue to dialog in the same way, how can we expect the outcome in our health or life circumstances to be any different?

In this instance, in these theories on attitude, and considering Khan's teaching, I am speaking in terms that "what we want to have happen, has already happened," as in healing. The thought or premise is to visualize what we want or desire to have happen in the here and now. Speak it as done and so it is. So, instead of praying for something we want, as an example, and asking for it to occur in the future, we expect it to happen in the here and now. We instead give thanks and praises to God or the Universe that it has already happened.

Attitude is a way of thinking, speaking, and acting as if everything is already accomplished. And so it is.

I walk by faith, not by sight

For many who have had health challenges—who are praying for something to occur and giving thanks later, or who have dealt with the constant nagging of negative thoughts or vibrations—this is going to be a new challenge for sure. Old habits, especially those deep in cellular memory, are going to be tough to break. To see it as already done, have the faith that God and the Universe have taken care of every detail (i.e., I am healed and with your spoken word it is done) in faith.

This sort of attitude adjustment will work with any scenario. All it takes is your faith, trust, and belief. Napoleon Hill, the author of *Think and Grow Rich,* put it this way: *"What the mind can conceive and believe it can achieve."* Change this to what the native being believes it can achieve, and you hit home. But, It is all attitudes!

We all need a little attitude adjustment sometimes, and now is a perfect time to start. It is done.

Chapter 36 –The Power of Words

The words we use & the power behind them

Today, since I understand the power of words and the energy behind them I will be aware of the words I use and convey only the messages that benefit the world and myself." - Parmahansa Yogananda.

"Words have much power." There is truth to that statement and people everywhere will profit by being conscious of the words they use and the energy they put behind them. It's in the energy behind the words that have a direct impact on our lives and the lives of all sentient beings...

Combine energy with the words used and we have power, whether in thought, written or spoken. We can box ourselves in by the words we use, or we can set ourselves free. How you ask? We do this by repeating words and phrases that decrease or increase our freedom and our ability to have the life we choose (i.e., good health, prosperity, and joy). What are the negatives that hold us down? You know them: *can't, won't, could have, would have, try, and not smart enough, not rich enough.* The list goes on and they are all essentially lies. With a change in attitude and words like "it is done" or "I am" used with intention, we can change our world. In any case, always turn polarity on the words that don't seem to work, or you will not have the outcome you desire.

Watch your words as they come out

Many people manage to get themselves into all kinds of therapies, treatments, exercise programs, diets, and healing modalities and emotional therapy sessions. We spend hours, months, years, and sometimes a lot of cash. Then we notice that things don't seem to have changed much! Why is this? What things can we do without that are holding things in place? WORDS! And the energy we put behind them.

I am not suggesting one go out and buy every book that was ever written on the subject of positive thinking, or attend seminars on "thinking your way to riches" or on healing for that matter. But the energy of thought, words, and actions or deeds certainly does shape our world.

Get rid of what you don't need

After clearing "unwanteds" (no such word? Oh no? Have you checked the top drawer of your dresser lately?), do a readjustment of attitude, and the words you use and what you have or what you bring into your lives can change substantially, now. Newly formed outflow will certainly be in order. Become conscious of the words you use and what you flow to the world and to people. If you are out flowing negative with the words you use on a regular basis to the same people all of the time, you are going to pick up agreements and power that help hold you in place. This is just what you do not want, and you will get the same result every time. I guarantee it. It is as true with speaking the words "it is done." And so it is. Speaking and acting in the positive will bring positive results. It is a physics matter and works every time when used cognitively.

Do this today

As an experiment, try to notice the words you use and your attitude (energy) behind them on a daily basis in each moment as you speak them. Be aware of the words you use, for the words you use and the energy behind them shape your world. Right? If you notice yourself using words that do not feel like they will have a beneficial outcome or the result that you intend, immediately pull the energy, pivot it, and reverse the outflow—turn polarity (a subject covered in an earlier chapter). Go to the exact time of the creation, and without any effort, simply spot the creation of words and emotions and reverse it—clear it. Replace it with **a new clear statement** of the original intention, not the mistaken outflow.

It may take more than just a few trials to get used to doing this but it's worth the time investment. Trust me on this one. It will change your world, including your health. This is the work of change, growth, and consciousness-raising many aspirants have been seeking for many years. If you want to change the world, change your attitude, and change your words. This is a progressive thing, and there is always some work to do. Unfortunately, most people don't even recognize the work or room for growth. Consider yourself BLESSED.

The words, intentions, and attitudes others use can have an effect on us as well. Become aware of flows coming to you that do not feel optimal. Use the same process. Go to the point of origin, the exact time of creation, and turn the flow (i.e., point of creation, turn polarity). Clear it until it's gone, and saying a simple "thank you" to the originator of the communication will do. Try not to use much effort or make more of a communication than what it is. When it's gone, *let it be gone without the need to re-create it,* whatever it was! It's sort of like never holding a grudge.

L. Ron Hubbard, the founder of Scientology and Dianetics, put it this way, "Decide on what you want, postulate it into existence in the here and now as though it is already done. Only now we must include allow the outcome to become your reality." There is no endorsement of Dianetics or Scientology made or intended here. I only used the quote to make a point. The only reason I use this quote is to help you, my reader, understand that YOU are in fact responsible for everything in your universe and in charge of your life destiny. When WE take responsibility for our own health and we do not expect a doctor, our parents, or lover, or a healer, or the government to be responsible for our health or well-being, we are in fact taking back our personal power to heal ourselves by the <u>words</u> we use and the postulates (energy) behind them.

I am well today. It is done!

More from my book *Open Spaces*

Every year in September at harvest time, The People come together for a Grass Dance to drum, dance, feast, and celebrate the abundance the Great Spirit has shared with the tribe. On the far eastern side of the "Res" there is a place known as the Sweetgrass Hills, named for a fair maiden who gave her life for unrequited love. Below these buttes lie the great plains of eastern Montana; and The People have gathered here for centuries on this ground, known as the common ground, where we come together in common good to dance and give thanks to the Creator for all his gifts.

This September was no surprise because it had a little of everything: hot air, warm showers, and heavy wind. Leonard used to tell me, "Don't come over here and cuss this wind because if you do, it will surely blow the roof right off my house," which is to say the wind blows a lot over the east.

The People love the Sweetgrass Hills for the Grass Dance. The grass reminds them of long ago, when it was knee high—long before the buffalo were gone and replaced by English cattle. They also appreciate being at the foot of one of the tribe's most sacred mountains. And the view to the west, back to the Rockies, is unbelievable.

Everyone is welcome at this event, although few non-Natives show up. It is not a Powwow, and there is no entertainment to speak of—no booths and no stick games or gambling. The People are there to give thanks for the gifts of life and to dance to the drum song in the sun.

It is no small gathering. Tribal folks from near and far come to attend. There are giveaways for good luck and some pretty good eating. It is a daylong event and most make a long drive home when it is over, as I did, because I had to be back in the office the following day. I made the drive home in three and one half hours that night.

The People gathered in large groups to hear the speeches of anyone that wished to speak or pray. These days the tribal leaders bring along a battery-powered loudspeaker so everyone can clearly hear the speaker, and no one is discouraged from talking.

When it was Leonard's turn to speak, he stood up and said, "O Great Spirit, you bring us many gifts. You give us our beautiful children, our homes, and plenty to eat, and we give thanks. You give us our women and the many gifts they bring to the men. We cherish these great gifts and the gifts to come. We see clearly that what we need, you provide us, and we give thanks. We feel deep in our hearts we are deserving of these blessings, and you continue to shower us with goods, with money, and with the clothes on our backs; and for this we know we are truly prosperous. We give thanks for our riches.

"We also know, Great One, that you like it when we are active in our accumulation of the goods we desire. We know that you are happy we have the faith and confidence to be abundant, based on what good we can do and what service we can be to our friends, family, and our Mother Earth. We feel your strength when we believe we are worthy of such great gifts and we allow them into our lives, and we give thanks. We gather today to give praise and thanksgiving for the gifts we have received, and we agree to allow even more goodness into our here-and-now experience. We agree to let our past be our past and move freely into this time of wondrous abundance and prosperity, and we give thanks for knowing we are also free and grand creators.

"Our hope, O Great One, lies in our faith and confidence in you, the Creator of all living things. We here today agree to give up worry because it only binds our hands from doing the works you see fit for us to do.

The People have many goals to accomplish and we know the work ahead of us. It does not worry us, for whatever we desire we know is done right here, right now, in your name, and we give thanks and praises. We now surrender the past to you and know it is the past. We are in great expectation of all the great gifts to come for all The People.

"We feel your presence and know that we are one with the Great Spirit and we give thanksgiving. We agree to have the courage to move through our days with wonder and excitement. We know that true joy is in the experience of being here to share with our loved ones and we place no importance on what we own, for it is only transitory. Our permanence lies in our love. *Ah U Hop Vista Doogie Vista Doogie Ah He.* Thank you for this day."

All The People shook their heads in agreement and everyone yelled out a big THANKSGIVING.

I learned from Leonard to be truly thankful. We do not have to wait for riches or great fortune to be thankful. If we look around us, we have plenty to be thankful for right now. How can we continually ask for more blessings when we do not give thanks for what has already been given to us?
O Great One and Leonard, I can never thank you enough.

In deep gratitude. Thank you.

Chapter 37 – Laugh It Out

Let's lighten it up a bit from my book *Miracles in the Kitchen.*

Laugh it out

There is nothing like a good joke to help lighten the load. In our enlightenment, there is the word lighten and not a bad word to include in our daily exercise in healing. Lighten up!

How many blondes does it take to change a light bulb? Never mind. You heard that one, I am sure; and the rest of my jokes are not clean enough to offer here. Please no mad blonde letters. That is just what I am talking about—lighten up.

How can you reduce the levels of chronic stress in your life and in your body and extend your lifespan, boost your immune system function, protect your nervous system and your sanity, and give your endocrine system a much-needed rest? Fortunately, there are several easy ways to do this. Let's look at the easiest one: laughter.

> You don't have to live in doubt. You can live in the secure knowledge of what is; and God, who is the great I AM, will bring that knowledge into being. And so it is!

There well may be more truth to this than one might tend to think at first thought. Is it possible that laughter actually has an effect on the human body in the same way that some medicines do? That is an interesting thought.

In truth, laughter helps to relieve stress, lighten pain, changes one state of mind, and can bring about spontaneous healing.

Laughter as therapy

There is real therapeutic value to laughter: to relieve stress, combat disease, and strengthen the immune system. Laughter no longer raises medical doubts. The idea that humor is healthy and that a hearty laugh can make a person feel much better has gained plenty of medical respectability in the last 20 years or more. The Dalai Lama himself is a great jokester.

Numerous research studies conducted in the West have led to the acceptance of laughter therapy. The case of Hunter "Patch" Adams (immortalized by actor Robin Williams in the film *Patch Adams*), who developed laughter therapy over 35 years at the Gesundheit! Institute in Virginia, USA is well known.

The other is the story of Norman Cousins, which is worth reading. The late editor of the American paper, *The Saturday Review*, took ill with ankylosing spondylitis, a severe connective tissue disease where the body just wastes away. When doctors gave up on him, he cured himself with large doses of vitamin C and comedies starring the Marx Brothers. Cousins found that ten minutes of belly laughter had an anesthetic effect and gave him at least two hours of pain-free sleep. He wrote about his experiences on self-healing through laughter in a best-selling book, *Anatomy of an Illness*.

This has been a book of inspiration for many practitioners of laughter therapy, including Dr. Madan Kataria, a Mumbai-based general practitioner who has pioneered the concept of laughter clubs in India. As founder of Laughter Club International, Dr. Kataria initiated over 300 laughter clubs all over India. Each of these conducts regular group laughter sessions on the premise that laughter is healthy for the spirit, body, and mind.

We still know very little about what happens in a person when we laugh, but there's a fair amount of evidence to suggest that laughter has wide-ranging effects on us psychologically and physiologically. The most obvious effect is on our mood, but laughter also keeps away negative emotions like anger, anxiety, and depression, which can tend to weaken the immune system. It relieves stress, a common cause of heart and blood pressure problems. Laughter improves lung capacity and oxygen levels in the blood and thus alleviates complaints of asthma and bronchitis. It also releases endorphins, the body's natural painkillers, thus reducing the frequency and intensity of arthritic pain and muscular spasms. It also helps with insomnia, migraines, allergies, and ulcers.

French neurologist Henri Rubenstein said that even one minute of laughter gives the body up to 45 minutes of therapeutic relaxation and healing of chronic illnesses. It can also reduce the heart rate and stimulate appetite and digestion.

French doctor Pierre Vachet, who studied the physiology of laughter, has stated that laughter expands the blood vessels and sends more blood racing to the extremities. As it sends more oxygen to every cell in the body, it also serves to speed tissue healing and stabilize many body functions. Other experiments have shown how watching funny films lowers our blood pressure and generates more endorphins in the blood, producing a feeling of health and well-being.

Many people who use laughter as therapy search for new jokes to read and pass on daily, stating that, "it just makes me feel better" to laugh and pass on good humor.

Another study in the late 1990's of patients recovering from surgery in a Florida hospital showed that the group allowed to choose the humorous movies benefited the most from laughter therapy and required fewer painkillers compared with a control group that saw none at all. A third group that was force-fed comedies without their consent or liking did the worst of all. This indicates that it is not something that can be force-fed, but rather by choice, one can in fact laugh one's self well.

It is clear that the idea that laughter or happiness is the best medicine is rapidly catching on. The British government in fact is proposing to hire comedians as jesters for the sick and the elderly. America also accepts humor as a legitimate input for management education. Apparently, some American companies such as IBM even have a humor adviser attached to the company to help keep a nice environment, help increase creativity, and increase productivity.

Other researchers in the USA have also established a close connection between humor and creativity. Since creativity requires playfulness—toying with words, ideas, pictures, and people—it interconnects with humor. Experts say that people who are afraid to play and who feel guilty about having fun and sharing a laugh rarely come up with creative new ideas. Even management guru Edward de Bono has observed that solutions to problems sometimes come through humor. Now, many doctors are beginning to agree with him. *Anatomy of an Illness*

A good friend of mine who lives here in Ojai had cancer several years ago. Her doctors told her she had only a short time to live and she should get her personal business in order. Essentially, she was to prepare for the worst.

Margaret refused to accept this news and went on to do her own research into what might help extend her life past the date given. She came across news of laughter therapy in an article she read in *Whole Life Times* and decided, well, this couldn't hurt.

While she did change her diet completely, and had extensive energy treatments aimed at pulling the entity cancer, she asserts a daily dose of good humor is what saves her. She watches old comedy movies, tunes into the comedy channel on TV, and reads a good joke every day. Now, has this saved her life? The only one who can decide on that is Margaret.

I have had chronic back pain since I was a boy. In my youthful ignorance, I was an accident waiting to happen and have broken 16 bones in 6 terrific accidents; which, actually there is no such thing because we all vibrate what we get.. In any case, my back has been a problem for me for several years. But, when one of my very best friends calls from back East all my pain disappears, he makes me laugh it out.

There are no adverse side effects from laughter. You may notice a change in symptoms, attitudes, and feelings, and there may be a few ups and downs. Don't get off the laughter kick too quick (hey, that rhymed). See Dave, we all have a little poet in us. Anyway, don't quit when you start to feel better. Continue it your whole life.

And yes, diet is important too

I am not for a moment suggesting that laughter alone will heal every challenge. Massage, energy manipulation, foods, diet, cleansing, exercise, and natural supplements are still very much in order, and one should not discount or stop their use just to laugh themselves into good health.

Foods that contain more enzymes of nature convert most easily into the body. And green foods are the material equivalent of good health and vitality. Combine with them, laughter.

Green and red vegetables are the finest products available for a healthy body. They give one sparkle to the eyes, glow to the skin, and immunity to the cells. Examples of green foods are whole, fresh, dark green and red organic vegetables and fresh, sweet, juicy fruits. Examples of foods that are not so great for healing are red meat, "junk" food, and canned, processed, packaged, or frozen foods. These types of foods are difficult to digest and are not supportive of the immune system. You want to eat foods that are alive, not dead. Rather than looking at the caloric content of food, first make sure it is lively with nature's brilliance. Food and laughter combined make for a healthy life (gee, new title for a new book).

There was a man who just won the lotto. He walked into a bar and there were two women sitting at the end of the bar…Oh, never mind. You probably heard it. But you get the idea I am sure.

Chapter 38 –Handling Negativity

Handling the illusion of Negativity is more apropos~ , since we go into agreement with the flow of negativity and judge it as real it is.

As discussed in an earlier chapter, using the phrase "mind, quiet" to handle negativity requires both processing and practice in life lessons out in the world. It requires one to recognize habitual negativity of the mind, cellular negativity of the body and aura, and resistance to negative outcome. By the being (person) him/herself to positively overcome or get through the habitual process of running around in circles that create the same or similar outcomes in our lives.

It's similar to being on a Mobius Strip; when a human being acts like a creature similar to a mouse and just keeps running the same figure eight pattern, not knowing why it does not get anywhere. Little does the poor mouse understand it is in the same place all the time because that is where it thinks it belongs. The only way to break this bond of negativity is through processing, and one can do this virtually on their own, by spotting the problem and turning polarity on it.

As with the mind, habitual negative thinking is a wonderful thing to waste. It serves no purpose other than possibly to make wrong an opponent or validate one's hidden desire to fail or remain stuck. If one were to change this phenomenon, they just might be free to take responsibility for succeeding at what they truly desire.

Habitual negativity, like other charges we have covered throughout this book, is locked somewhere in the body and aura. Either a practitioner or the individual themselves can find it, call it up, and turn and release this stuff.

Remember now, this is all about processing, and life is a process. Getting closer to Godhood is a process, so finding this charge and releasing it all at once may not be possible. After all, you have had six billion years to create it, so it just may not go away over night. Nevertheless, one can expect miracles and experience them. I have seen this a thousand times.

The places in one's body to start hunting this charge

Start by balancing the Chakras and running healing light up and down the body—in, through, and out. Pick your favorite color, or the favorite color of your client, and run that color through the body. Continue until the body FEELS cool and relaxed as possible.

When things FEEL pretty much in order and you are ready to hunt this "little devil" down, look for it contained in, on, or around the body. Call up statements containing "loser," "can't," "won't," "shouldn't," "couldn't," and "wouldn't." Find thoughts of "conceiving achievement" and locate the counter thought that contains "fail." Here is an easy example:

"I think I will go to the grocery store and pick up a few things."

Oh but there may not be any place to park. This is after all the busiest time of the day. I better stay home and wait till later. Bingo! A negative thought just caused one to give up on going to the grocery store. Right there we need to run "point of creation, turn polarity"—turn

262

polarity throughout all time, all space, all dimensions—release, and disconnect. Replace it with, "Oh, I think I will go to the store now!"

Have you seen this? Have you ever noticed people whose lives just don't seem to be going well? Do you find that they often complain about how hard life is? I'm sure you've heard it. It goes something like this, "Oh, these damn kids! Oh hell, the electricity needs work! Damn old car won't start again! Did you hear that Alice has cancer? My boss just won't get off my back. If I just had more money, everything would be okay. The economy is falling apart. The roof is caving in, and oh, my goodness, those poor people in Africa (not that there are not poor people in Africa)" But this person refuses to find anything positive going on in their lives, has little or no creativity, and will actually try to curtail creativity whenever it raises its "ugly threatening head."

Where is this coming from?

- The mind
- Cellular memory
- Habitual negativity

The challenge for a practitioner is to go in, with the willingness of the client, find the charge connected to this stuff, and clear it and work to set the client on a new path of positive postulates. This will take resolve on both the client's and the practitioner's part to help create a new life scenario.

Negativity subjects and where to find them

How many negative thoughts, ideas, considerations or

projections are not beneficial to our ultimate outcome in life? Geese, why not ask how many thoughts are there? There are thousands per day!

While the list may be endless, the process remains the same. Handle them with "point of creation, turn polarity," release and disconnect, and replace them with a clear postulate of the original design or the desired outcome.
"I can't make it. It won't work. I might fail. What if it doesn't work?" The negative thought is never the original thought. The original thought comes from the creative life force and the second negative thought comes from hell. The enemy here is really just the mind, which can play hell on an individual and has for about six billion years.

How to spot negative thoughts, feelings, and emotions is just to allow oneself to experience it, allow it to come up, and then turn it. This is among our biggest hurdles as humanoids. As a practitioner you will spot this stuff in your client by the way it feels—very heavy until turned—and then there is no sensation at all.

Where is this stuff in or on the body? Run you hands over it until you find it. Look deeply into the heart Chakra, solar plexus chakra, root and third eye.

Run it out till it clears

Run[29], find, and turn polarity on negativity every day for the rest of your life with this stuff, because it is there. It

[29]   Run means to do the process, find the charge, and relieve the cause.

lays hidden but nevertheless it is there; and when you clear it, you are off the roof and flying.

When was the last time you wanted to ask for a raise, but didn't? How many times have you thought about asking someone out on a date but changed your mind because you were certain the answer would be no? How many times have you stopped yourself from becoming an artist or great writer? How many times have you just wanted to say what you felt to your spouse or boss and couldn't because you thought the outcome would be disastrous just because something in your head said, "No, don't try, or I am not good enough"? I'm not talking about inner intuition. I'm talking about a creation that you wanted and then turned your back on because that little voice said, "No don't try it, or you will fail." That is the negativity we, after all, hear. Always speak from the heart, and you will soon, just after this polarity is turned and released.

How many people in the world do you know who have the ability to clean up our planet's drinking water but refuse to try? How many people have had a great idea for a new invention but would not take a risk because they might lose? How many businesses, charities, schools, or children would be served if we didn't have this little machine in place that said, "No, don't try"? Could world peace be just around the corner? Yes, and it is.

Take these negative emotions, thoughts, vibrations, considerations, and ideas. Turn polarity on them, then go out, and create a whole new world. I know you can do it!

Handling negativity will do just that in our own lives, and

for our governments, churches, mosques, and schools. And so it is…

Chapter 39 –Spirituality and Healing

In God It Is Done and so it is...

It has been said in many ways and many times; God Is All There Is.
The truth in that statement runs deep; it is a spiritual belief for millions of people worldwide. The commonality of faith in God/Goddess is as basic as air and a way of life for many metaphysical people as well as Hindu's Christians, Jews, Muslims and Pagans alike.

The basic thought principle has remained in place for many, many years-God Is All There Is; The All In All. Found in ancient text of the Egyptians, Greeks, Celtics and Native indigenous people throughout the world. "There is nothing but God" or God is all there is. The principle speaks of God's love, Gods joy, Gods goodness that lives in each one of us and that God is good and lavish abundance, in health, wealth and long life. In Gratitude it is done is the theme of the day.

The truth that God/Goddess lives within us has a long standing tradition of "let go and let God" and when we do, soulful things happen in our lives in terms of perfect heath, perfect mate, perfect home, perfect wealth, perfect harmony and peace. This truth has not changed and may never as it could be as close to an absolute as we may find.

What can tend to foul thinks up for humanoids are #1 forgetting and two illusions. Forgetting is considered one of the major fumbles for all humanoids, because in forgetting we give up our Native` knowingness of who we truly are. Illusions are energies that can get us fouled up and lock us out of living a God righteous life. While these illusions feel and seem very real, they can all be handled by remembering—remembering who we are and allowing our oneness with God/Goddess *within* to guide our lives. In God all things are perfect all of the time, and so it is.

When and where necessary there are in fact scientific/metaphysical practices that will in fact assist humanoids in their quest for full unfoldment of the soul and being (living as Gods) that we all are. The materials above should have covered this completely.

In God it is already done...

In practice we can in fact remove the barriers to total freedom and return to that which we truly are-Godself. By removing barriers, blocks, locks, considerations, conclusions, projections, judgments and a whole host of unwanted conditions, we come into the realization of that which we truly are, and live as Grand Glorious Creators in oneness with God/Goddess in perfect peace, harmony and joy and with all living Gods and Goddesses. In God it is done.

One day perhaps it could be done with a snap of a finger, but for now humanoids enjoy the game and the challenge, the work of waddling ourselves out of the maze to find (see or *feel*) God within and allow our lives to be the experience of perfection, we deserve.

Occasionally we require assistance, a healing and a breaking free from such blocks. Everything is perfect all of the time and so it is In Truth everything is perfect all of the time in God. Through meditation, visualization, relaxation and focus we come to find that God/Goddess does in fact live in the innermost tiniest place in our hearts as the very source of all life. Through **God's** breath of life we live in perfect love of God we live gloriously—everything is perfect all of the time.

Occasionally we need to process life's illusion and become free to live as grand glorious creators. There are however perfect natural embodied souls living in oneness as Gods/Goddesses here and now.

Humanoids have managed over the millenniums to foul things up pretty good, now the chore of clearing out the collection of Illusions/delusions and remembering has become the goal of many mankind, rising to Godkind in the true unfoldment of the soul. But it has become necessary to do the work and the work is that of removing the barriers to oneness and allowing the full unfoldment of the soul to occur-hence God realization.

This road, the path my seem bumpy at times as well it should be; we have managed to create quite an interesting game for ourselves and working through the maze of confusion--and out has become quite a chore for many humanoids.

But! Please don't forget the party. Lightened up! As it has been said by many prominent "Guru's." Enlightenment very much has to do with the party, with the dance and joy. Try to have some fun on the road or just stay home. I have always said, if in ain't fun I anin't goin. Yes, no doubt there is a time for reverence, there is a time for quiet contemplation, there is a time for processing energies. But, there must be a time for life, or it just plain is not fun. God wants this to be fun for you and me, he/she or she wants you to have a more pleasurable experience in this plane, and life is not

about suffering.
Come in to the unfoldment in Love Peace and Joy, and come to the party.

My Prayer for you: *God is light. God is love, divine right order, and prosperity. God is the earth, the sky, and beyond this universe. God is positive energy and light flowing through you, in, and around you. God is air and water, through me and you, right here and now. God is our thoughts, ideas, and mind ever expanding and extending into the visible and the invisible. God is all there is…*

I am whole in God.
I am health in God.
I am prosperity in God.
I am peace in God.
God is all there is.
I am LOVE in God.

God is the light that beams through me and out to others that call upon God-light. God is with me, in me, as you and me. We are one in God. We are whole, connected, and centered. God is forever loving me and guiding me to my highest level of good in life. I know He/She does the same for you and everyone in the Universe. God is truth and light every-where—north, south, east, and west. God is centered and connected to us all. God is in us all, around us all, and loves us all. God is all there is. He/She is divine love, prosperity with me, and everyone here and now.

I know that I am, and everyone is, living our divine path, in divine right order. God manifests Himself in our hearts, souls, and minds through love. He desires people, plants, and animals to be in perfect health and harmony in the here and now.

God's plants, Goddess's Earth, and God's people are forever protected and provided for, so graciously He/She loves us. We connect with One-ness and God lives in the peaceful vibration of us all.

God Lives in me and as He/She does you.

Our fruits of labor are in our realization in the here and now. God's seed is planted and growing into us now. We are healed and whole.
We love to help and be of service to others. We are blessed with peace, love, prosperity, and joy in our service.

God is love. God loves us and nurtures us by that spirit. Our ancestors and angels knew and know of this; and we do as well today, and so it is.
We are blessed. We are in the divine right order. God delivers blessings to every person at the right time. The doors of opportunity open wide and flow with abundance of success, knowledge, good health, prosperity, and money. All is so good!!
We are Love, Peace, and Joy in Unity. In God

I am so grateful that God/Goddess is allowing the living of my dreams, desires, and wishes that God/Goddess has given to me; and I am so grateful that God/Goddess is also living for my dreams, desires, and wishes that He/She has given to me. Thank you, Great Spirit, for the wonderful lives and blessings that you have for all of us.

With this awareness, I simply release the truth to the Law of the universal truth and let go and know it is

271

done!!! And so it is.

Aum-AMEN

There is truth in prayer and positive affirmation. The truth is in you.

She never gave up her faith

A friend of mine had started college right after high school, as is usually the norm. Shortly after the start of her freshman year, her aunt passed away and left three children, one of them in his early teens, one of them in the last years of being a child, and one of them a mere baby of two. Although she was by no means old enough to be "mother" to the oldest two, my friend left school. By working together, the four of them managed to help the severely disabled father of this family hold the family together.

My friend never regretted doing this, and went on to a specialized school when she was older, but she often wondered what she would have done in a "regular" college or university. Forty something years later, she found herself living in a small college town, assisting some people who were mentally challenged with their independent living. The local college, a very highly esteemed privately-owned institution, offered the opportunity for older people to take some non-credit "enrichment" classes which were peer taught for a nominal amount of money, and so my friend signed up for them.

Although the classes were interesting, they weren't what my friend wanted, and one day the thought came to her, "I'm going to graduate from that college." With no money available other than her Social Security Disability check that she received monthly for having been struck by a car a number of years earlier, which had left her as a wheelchair user, my friend went into the registrar's office and asked about becoming a student at the college. She came out the highest achieved freshman. She never gave up her faith in herself and Goddess's support in everything she did.

Not only did my friend graduate from the college, but also she graduated with honors and as a member of a prodigious honor society. My friend also received honors for being in the top one percent of all of the college and university students in the United States for two years in a row. The amazing thing, at least by sight, is that the entire four-year education didn't cost my friend a single cent. In fact, she made money on the deal.

My dear friend knew that there was no way that she could afford to attend this college, yet she also knew what God said about Himself, that with Him, all things are possible, and that He gives us the desires of our hearts. So she stepped out in faith and took God at His word—the same word you hear today that leads you to your own highest good.

God has these same sorts of blessings for all of us, not just for my friend. God is our prosperity, peace, long life, and good health. Quiet yourself and just listen, and breathe God's words in. If we look at the natural world and say, "I can't," we probably will be right; but if we look at God and say, "I can. Through Him, I can do all things," we will be right in that also. When we find something that we want very much to do, the question isn't, and "Can I do this?" The question is, "How am I going to do this?" There is a big difference. A positive affirmation holds truth and helps guide our way.

If you focus on solutions instead of problems, and enlist God's help, the solutions come to you.

Each one of us has dreams. You can't measure Dreams according to the world's standards. You measure Dreams strictly in regard to the importance they have to the individual. What might seem like a small dream to one might be a big dream in the life of someone else. Dare to dream big concerning the things that are important to you. Don't take someone else's measuring stick to your dream. Measure it only by what it means to you. Take that dream to God in prayer and know that He/She, in whom you are whole; He/She, in whom you have perfect health; He/She, who will provide you with prosperity; He/She, who is your peace; and He/She, who is everywhere and in all, will answer your prayer.

There <u>is always something to pray about (process).</u> This is life on planet Earth and beyond. In the process, I wish you Love, Peace, and Joy.
In Oneness with God/Goddess, we find our true home.

Chapter 40 – Cracking the DNA Code

Many philosophers have postulated ideas on longevity and living a long, healthy life for several hundred years in this recent history, but to be more exact, in truth, for millions of years, here on planet Earth or elsewhere we have sought a life of longevity and deathlessness. The main question is, "How long can we live?" Can we crack The DNA Code[30] and live forever? Some philosophers and scientists are currently researching to a very deep level to explore and investigate the immortality of men and women, while many spiritualists might agree that we are, after all, immortal beings and we truly never die.

That is fine for the infinite souls! However, what about the body? How long can it go on? Is Enoch or Christ actually walking around in the same body they have always had? Have they so completely realized their native One-ness with God/Goddess that they never "died"?

Further, the computation/postulate exists that with enough personal control, awareness, and personal power (i.e., our realization of who we really are—God or pure consciousness), we can live forever. "*Once we arrive at the "knowingness" of who we truly are, we shall not perish, but live forever.*" Ras[31].

Is living forever possible? Many believe it is so. Many

---

[30]   The DNA Code is a wrapped, in-capsulated implant that contains a death postulate.
[31]   Ras refers to Rasputin, an entity known to many Rasputin seekers of truth.

of our greatest thinkers, writers, and philosophers in so-called new age paradigms, quantum physics, applied religious philosophies, and science agree on the principle of the power of intention, decisions, and original thought. In truth, original thought has much power in our lives and as to how long we live. That is, there is the notion that we are the creators of our own original thought and that with enough awareness, personal power (energy), concentration, or focus, we certainly do have the power to live a very long time, even indefinitely.

Also important to the equation are Matter, Energy, Space, and Time, with energy being the controlling factor. I will get more into this with the message that follows below. Suffice to say, by controlling certain energy flows we can live for a length of time heretofore thought impossible.

In order to comprehend the material discussed within this document, understanding cellular memory processing is essential. Please note that I have explained in detail cellular memory processing, including energy flows and pivoting energy, throughout the second part of this book. To understand this background information, it is essential that one re-reads, understands, and applies the methods in the aforementioned chapters.

For those of you who are reading this document and who read my earlier publication on the DNA Code, please be aware that it is essential to understand these processes completely. Take the time to go back through the earlier material and really get it. Questions will certainly come up during the reading of this material: What about a body that just gives up? What about obtaining a new, younger body (if one considers reincarnation as real)? Questions like this will arise: Do you mean people can survive terminal cancer, heart disease, or a tragic accident? Yes to all of the above.

One may assert that one does not wish to live forever, and that is perfect too, as we all have personal power, so we have personal choices. We all make choices every day in our lives, in all areas, including death and dying.

There seems to be some power outside ourselves that we align with and give power to. That is the power of attachment and detachment. These are in-capsulated[32] implants. It appears that we should not have any connection to either. That is, if we want to go on living for a very long time or forever for that matter, attachment/detachment must be a cleared factor. The contemplation of attachment versus detachment can have an equally significant impact on other areas of our lives, such as money, health, Love, purpose, and so on. Ras covers this completely. *In summary, he advises that we let go of our attachments and detachments.*

One can run this process of letting go of our attachments and detachments and expect to feel healthier, more vital, and a returned sense of purpose. Revitalizing basic purpose gives one enough power to "wake the dead." The natural outcome to running this process of letting go of our attachments and detachments to death and dying can increase one's longevity, or living forever, as one chooses.

The following is research partially based on channeled

---

[32]   in-capsulated refers to the smallest of the cells, a hidden and egg-shaped cell. Its purpose is to make less of.

information from the entity Ras, or Rasputin, to be more exact. Ras came to me to deliver this message. Other thoughts have come from a few other contributing entities, and some are my own conclusions. I hope you find this material valuable and are able to put it to good use in your life and in the lives of those you LOVE.

Channeled information from Ras

Dear Ones,

Humans can crack these codes to unlock the mystery and the apparent need to die or give up the body. The codes, in fact, do unlock the keys to life and the dying of the human body. The codes are contained at the very smallest cellular level and are hidden within in-capsulated cells that contain decisions, conclusions, contracts, postulates, projections, judgments, agreements, resistances, and fear of death and dying.

This information you are about to receive is, in fact, at the very deepest level of awakening and for those seeking a deep understanding of who they truly are and regaining their personal strength and power. It will prove itself valuable in its application "for information without application is useless."

People of planet called Earth desire various things, among the stuff they consider important. One may consider money, homes, cars, trucks, SUVs, and other toys to be of extreme value and importance in one's life, and I have no judgment on what one possesses or does not create to possess. If money brings one happiness in some

278

form, whatever form, I am happy for one.

In truth, one most desires LOVE. People of planet Earth desire Love, Peace, Joy, Freedom, Knowledge, Wisdom, and the return to knowing who they truly are and exactly what they have come here to do. People require of themselves to live in harmony with others and the return to the knowingness of one spirit, no matter how one labels it.

Channeled

We Are One—individual but one!
In this opportunity to unravel the DNA Codes, one shall find the keys to true peace, happiness, joy, and LOVE. One will also learn how to apply them in their lives.

Jay, in summary, if one just breathes and relaxes, one shall possess all of the knowledge by oneself. There is a practical application one could DO on a daily basis that will bring one to exactly where one wishes to be. Be it enough to say just "breathe."
Ras

Information from Ras and Mother

Breathe. Take in Goodness's (if one should judge such) fresh, clean mountain air. Breathe in through your nose completely. Inhale goodness, knowledge, wisdom, peace, joy, harmony, and LOVE completely. Exhale all toxins through your mouth. Let out all poisons, lies, evil (if one should judge such). Also, let go completely of all attachments—detach from the world and relax.

279

Exhale and relax.

Just Breathe

Continue to breathe. Continue daily to consciously breathe and relax. For several minutes every day, just breathe and allow what you most desire to come into your experience, enter into your sphere, and appreciate it in whatever form it comes in, with no judgment of the experience. Give thanks.

Breathe, relax, and allow. It does not matter what you allow into your experience as long as you most desire it: long life, health, peace, joy, harmony, creation, destruction of evil. Break away and *pivot* your attachment to decisions, conclusions, projections, judgments, fears, angers, regrets, contracts, postulates, and all attachment to resistance to what you think you do not want. Just breathe, relax, and allow. Allow the experience of your own choosing and experience it completely. Allow the result you desire to occur, without attachment to it, and relax.

"Too simple," one may say. "I can't just breathe myself into living a long life or forever. It's just not scientifically possible!"

"No," says Ras. "Okay, let's go deeper into relaxation." Throughout one's many incarnations, one has departed from One-ness many times and gives up or refuses to know who they truly are. One may be implanted with thoughts, ideas, projections, judgments, considerations, decisions, conclusions, resistances, fears, and unknowingness. This has only helped to decrease one's ability to know and one's own personal power to choose one's life experience here on planet Earth. At the very deepest level, held IN[33] by one's own power through focus and resistance, one has decreased one's ability to live a very long time or forever.

To break the DNA Code, one must breathe, relax, and pivot the energy connected to the Code. By pivoting, we mean turning polarity enough to where all resistance dissipates, and there is no charge (energy) left on the subject.

One who has departed from One-ness has left the Sun. They separate them self from universal knowledge and GOD/GODDESS power. They refuse to Know. That, my dear ones, is how one dies—by giving up one's own power, strength, and abilities.

Break the DNA Code

Find the implant on a cellular energy level contained within in-capsulated form. Pivot the thought, idea, judgment, attachments, detachments, conclusions, and resistance on the original postulate that one cannot live forever, one must die. Turn polarity, pivot the energy, and allow it to dissipate and then release and disconnect completely. By disconnecting, one disconnects themselves from the agreement and the resistance to connect to the thing itself. Releasing and disconnecting are essential.

As in all procedures in this book, there is a procedure to unlocking the DNA Codes, and finally here it is. One may run this procedure on oneself, also apply it to others, and help to relieve their suffering from dis-ease and death, and turn polarity on the requirement for one's body death experience.

[33]   IN means held in, as in trapped.

Here is the procedure:

From Ras:
> *In Mother/Father God, join in unison with us here today. Guide us into our highest state, and let us be one with you. Shroud us in light, protection, and LOVE. Give us the wisdom to be what you would have us be.* Very Good. Let us begin, Ras.

Breathe, relax, and allow

Take three deep breaths, inhale completely, and exhale completely. And relax! Inhale all goodness. Exhale all toxins. Relax and allow yourself to be the divine creator that you are (we are all divine creators of our own experience). Allow perfect health, longevity, perfect peace, LOVE, joy, and abundance into our experience. And so it is...

DNA implant open

Give the instructions "DNA implant open" to oneself or to another's self. Relax and locate the original postulate. That is, locate the time, place, form, and event of the idea that one must die or give up one's body, according to DNA implant. Find the thought, conclusion, decision, agreement, and resistance to death. Turn polarity (pivot) on the energy connected to the original postulate. Turn it completely throughout all time, all space, and all dimensions. Turn the original thought or idea about death and dying. On a DNA level, turn polarity, release, and disconnect. Disconnect from the attachment of the outcome and breathe. Continue until all charge dissipates. Run your hands over your body to find the in-capsulated charge. Pull it out and send it elsewhere (See the chapter on Cellular Memory Processing).

Once complete, stop! Run the procedure until all charge dissipates. When it's done, it's done, and it's time to move on.

Now, repeat the following mantra for yourself or a loved one:

> *I am a grand creator. I choose my longevity. I choose life and my good health. I break all contracts, agreements, and decisions on or about death and dying. I choose life and so it is.*

One will find this energetic DNA charge hidden within in-capsulated form. One must defuse the capsule and release the charge, allow it to go, and allow oneself to be reborn into a new original postulate by regaining one's ability to set new postulates and therefore live as long as one chooses or not. In truth, there is no death. There is only life with new beginnings.

Implanted commands and phrases to look for defuse the capsule and unlock the charge, thus cracking the codes:

Run these codes, commands, and phrases and any others you find:[34]
- *I am going to die some day.*
- *I can't spot DNA Code.*
- *I am afraid to die.*
- *Fear of death.*
- *Everybody dies.*

---

[34] "Run these commands and phrases and any others you find" means to process them to completion so there is no charge remaining.

- *I just can't take this. I want to die.*
- *We all die.*
- *It is in my DNA that I am going to die.*
- *No one lives forever.*
- *Dying is just part of the deal.*
- *Two things you can depend on are death and taxes.*
- *No one is immortal.*
- *The body just does not live forever.*
- *I am getting too old to live much longer.*
- *The body ages and dies. That is how things work.*
- *I was created to die.*
- *The game is a trap. Everyone dies in the end.*
- *The body is like a machine that just breaks down and dies.*
- *I am dying here.*
- *I am dying.*
- *Death is inevitable.*
- *No one lives past 110 years old.*
- *You can expect to die at about the same age as when your parents did.*
- *I do not want to live past (a predetermined age).*
- *The body withers and dies.*
- *Who wants to live in an ill body?*
- *DNA implant forced upon one by mother.*

The above codes, implants, instructions, phrases, and commands are examples of what one may find hidden in the codes of GE/DNA[35]. If you run these and others and you will find a point of no charge. Then set in place in your own universe a new postulate—by your own

---

[35]   "GE" means Genetic Entity Code, the code apparently passed on by one's parents.

choice.

People can run these procedures on themselves by closing their eyes, breathing, relaxing, and sweeping their own hands over their body to help locate where the charge is, pull it out, and turn polarity (pivot) the energy.

Practitioners, use this procedure to run the implants off using your hands three to four inches over your client's body in the same fashion as all other processes. This may take more than one session to get all of this charge. There are millions of years of accumulated charge to get, so get it all. The outcome is improved health, vitality, returned or renewed purpose, and, of course, longevity.

Run the process more than once per lifetime, as this stuff can "key-in" or become active from just walking down the street. For this reason alone, apply breathing techniques daily and relax. The above procedure does not require power or force. Use it gently, effortlessly, and with total ease and joy. Just breathe and allow.

One will find DNA Code charges hidden in the GE force as well. One will use the same procedure as above for unlocking GE/DNA Code. Locate the original postulate as a being coming into life (a body) postulating death and run source (original postulate), POCTP[36]. Release and disconnect from this charge in the same manner as above. They are, in fact, two separate but equal implants[37]. What is the important ingredient is that we defuse the energy from the original postulate (implant) and regain our own personal strength and power back,

---

[36]   POCTP means point of creation, turn polarity.
[37]   Implants refer to ideas, considerations, postulates, and so on that are forced in and held in place by agreement or resistance.

allowing one to easily control matter, space, and time, and the ability to use our energy to be the most fun.

Note to practitioners: Find the original postulate and turn polarity by using your hands, as in all procedures throughout this book.
Of curious notation is the "is-ness" (is what it is) that we get, what we get, from implants by either accepting (agreeing with) them, or to our own resistance to the same. One chooses their longevity with clarity. One can remain with one's body indefinitely.

Questions for Ras

Do you mean we just locate the time we decided to die on a DNA level, turn polarity on it, and live forever?

Ras: Yes!

What about good health practices on planet Earth? Are they real or not?

Ras: These are merely considerations, but yes, your friend Jay wrote a whole book devoted to good eating practices, diet, exercise, and good health. One may choose to read it. Find Jay's book *Miracles In the Kitchen* at his website www.OneGlobePress.com and download it. Yes, among the choices you make are what you ingest.

How do I know if I have found the original postulate?
Ras: You will know by how it *feels*. If it's "hot," stay with it until it cools and dissipates completely.

What if I get sick or something and don't want to live forever?
Ras: Choices, my friend. It is all about choices. Run "getting sick" with the same procedure as above.

How are my happiness, joy, and purpose connected to longevity?
Ras: Your happiness depends on you discovering who you really are and living what you came here to do, not on how long you keep your present body.

Is the aging process included in this process?
Ras: Yes, run the same exact process with the aging command as the implant phrase to pivot, such as, "Everybody gets old, or we all age."

You mentioned in the beginning processing all areas of our life with this data. Can you expand on this?
Ras: Yes, everything in one's life has polarities. Pivoting is essential in order for one to break free of the chains that bind one. Please read Jah Jay's book *Open Spaces*. He covers other areas completely and with harmony in nature.

Chapter 41 – In Conclusion: The Final Destiny

We have certainly come a long way from simple massage for relaxation purposes, haven't we? But reaching for enlightenment and the unfoldment of the soul in fact does require deep relaxation.

While massage alone will not assist one in achieving the ultimate destination, it does help pave the way and put the seeker of truth on the path with ease and less distraction, for it is distraction alone that pulls one off the path and away from the goal.

In the last several chapters we covered "turning polarity" and releasing discomfort, anxiety, loss, grief, anger, fear, worry, doubt, deep-seated long held onto postulates, considerations, enforced or implanted realities, less than sane postulates and conclusions, and disallowed power, and so on. Do not discount or push aside this methodology lightly. This will help one to achieve freedom from an overzealous mind. It will also assist one in finding out who they truly are and regain the ultimate Source.

It starts with the very light and easily accessible chains locked in, on, and around the body (cells), mind, and spirit. We addressed what needed to be addressed first, which is not to fix anyone but to clear away debris and open one to the higher states of consciousness available when one starts to look deeply, and to clear away millenniums of debris—thoughts, ideas, considerations, conclusions, decisions, counterproductive ideas, agreements, resistances, judgments, and projections.

We can start with communication issues, abilities, and disabilities in this area. Then turn polarity enough to where one gains complete personal control to communicate on any level, anywhere, anytime, on any subject. Then we can proceed on, moving one through a series of processes to peel the onion to get to the core, so to speak, and do processes that hold one back from the goal, and finally have the ultimate release. Knowing.

We then move to problem solving, which is finding the true source for all perceived problems. We work to relieve all suffering, remove all anger, hostility, and upsets with self, others, groups, tribes, and so on, so that one comes to recognize his/her One-ness with all living things. We clear away all blocks to one's ability to be in their personal power and never disparage it. We clear one to assist in finding true clarity and "Being-ness," which is in total One-ness with all sentient beings and to be in perfect allowance without the need for opposition whether created, resisted, or forced upon. We move to opposition processing, which clears the mind and allows one to move up the grade into unfoldment with ease and joy.

Finding Love, Peace, and Joy in ourselves and all creatures

When we find ourselves stabilized in a renewed spirit and have achieved direct communication with our higher self, we then are able to move on to what are considered to be the higher realms, or perhaps more esoteric stages of the unfoldment of who we are, where we came from, why we are here, and the final destination—realization and unfoldment of the soul.

Endless processing

There is no doubt today that processing can appear to be endless; but alas, there is finality. What many have come to realize is that it has taken us billions of years to get where we are. If we are to experience Joy, Peace, and Love in harmony with all creatures from this planet and others, we just may have some work cut out for us to achieve the final destination—creativity.

Relax; it will not be a billion-year cycle to come to the goal

What distracts one from coming to the unfoldment is distractions and disharmony in body, mind, and spirit. Disharmony feels heavy, feels painful, feels like prison. Harmony feels like joy, glee, freedom, fun, pleasure, and enjoyment. One wants to be there and not feel fight-or-flight. Here, there is no truth to left brain/right brain thinking because there is no brain. That is merely an illusion.

Although the feeling of distraction may be necessary for one to cut the junk out or get through various barriers, one does not have to be in an endless processing in order to achieve harmony with self and all other living things.
Experience the distractions and disharmony. Process it, release it, disconnect, and never rebuild it again. This is tricky you see, because Homo sapiens love playing tricks on themselves. In this lies a very deep problem of never allowing freedom or reaching the goal, which is the ultimate freedom.

When one spots an area that the mind has focused on (charge built on a subject), one needs to process it.

Negativity must come off so the positive energy can come through and allow for the ultimate achievement of the goal. One does not have to spend one's life processing "it". One should be living life and leaving time for processing to say, three to four hours per day. If one walks in processing, one is missing the joy of the day. Don't pass by the sunset today to be processing yesterday. Be here now, and worry about tomorrow yet another day. In truth, never worry about tomorrow. Live now.

Twin and solo processing

The best way to do processing is with friends, exchanging time allotted for each to give and receive treatment. When one reaches a level of understanding that one is able to apply these techniques to themselves for their own benefit, one may solo process. Reports by many practitioners indicate that the one performing the treatment for another also receives benefit at the same time, which is to say, gets the same relief as the client.

One will have all the opportunity one wishes to process, relieve pain and discomfort, and to assist one to move up into higher knowingness. One will have the space, time, and facilities to help one recover all native abilities and beyond. Please try not to make this an endless process. You will find yourself in a constant search for, "What's wrong with me and how can I fix it?" This is a trap within itself. If one comes to this conclusion that one requires constant processing, one will stay trapped in the postulate for many lifetimes.

Run the surface processes first

Run all body problems first. That includes all aches,

pains, discomforts, illnesses, traumas, dramas, diseases, and imbalances. This may require concentrated effort in processing and lifestyle changes. Change in diet and exercise may come into the picture. One may choose a juice fast, a deep cleanse, sweating, acupuncture, massage, meditations, yoga, prayer or positive affirmations, vitamin supplements, or herbal remedies for specific challenges. The important factor here is a clear running body will assist one in the achievement of the goal—unfoldment—with ease.

One may come to a practitioner of the healing arts with many complaints. It is the practitioner's duty to find the outstanding issues—the most apparent problems— and deal with these first before attempting to take the aspirant to higher levels of understanding. Esoteric knowledge without applicability is useless, and one will not get it. After assisting one to overcome present distractions, the practitioner is then able to move on, assisting in turning other areas that will lead one to the final goal—total understanding.

As the practitioner recognizes shifts, improvements, added strength, and abilities in the client's consciousness and aura, then we can move the aspirant from relief of shadow self to handling influential beings from other planets and so on.

The work is about releasing and removing blocks and barriers that disallow one to live in perfect harmony with self and all living things. You accomplish this by lifting charge that entraps one in unhappiness, misery, insanity, ignorance, or a lack of joyfulness, fulfillment, and peace.

The methods used for this work always remain the

same. Changes in methodology come in as we open to higher self and awareness. There will come a day when all we must do is snap our fingers and needed changes will occur. For now, please use this method—point of creation, turn polarity, release and disconnect—until abilities shift.

Using our hands over the client's (aspirant's) body to locate charge and instructing such to turn polarity until it dissipates, and asking one to disconnect, is the simplest form we have for relieving barriers, blocks, and charge.

The more esoteric routes to freedom are not in any certain order but are run with the same method. All are made of matter, energy, space, and time. Remember this work is about dealing with energies and not the significances of the other three components.

Higher levels of release

Always search for implants, grids, worm holes, Galactic Monsters, destroyers, Mobius strips, holograms, self-concluded decisions to be unlocked, enforced realities, non–friendly entities, and all HEAD-centered considerations as listed above, "THE DEVIL," and other incarnation realities from here or elsewhere that cause one to NOT be here now. Remove all addictions. Relieve stress from the job, money, home life, parental influence, excluded from One-ness, can't be in a body/must be in a body, self-debased removal of personal power to control one's own universe, and inability to allow happiness and complete survival, including prosperity and abundance.

Collapse each item and ask the aspirant to disconnect,

draw back their personal energy and power, set a new decision in place, and allow that to be the governing factor in well-being, joy, happiness, peace, and Love in their lives now and forevermore.

Always search for the unacceptable, the unattainable, and the unknown. Check all chakras for all areas of upset and discomfort. Always end a session with renewing the client to re-newness, complete with new postulates.

Processing may appear to be endless. There is always some-**thing** to process that leads one away from the ultimate reality to knowing—knowing exactly who one is and the final realization of God/Goddess-hood.

Once we come to recognize who we are and that we are the source of our personal universe, that we are completely able to play this game on earth, we can win. "Win?" one asks. We can win at the game of finding our way out of the agreed upon or resisted game—*one must not know* implant. With the achievement of knowing, one comes to know "I am God" and so it is. Yes, game over, you win.

Here's an example:

When we break the ties that bind us into our own personal slavery, we are setting ourselves free to be the grand creators that we all are. It is the practitioner's responsibility to assist the aspirant in realigning with who they truly are—God.

When you reach a clean spot (i.e., an area of concern or charge you helped to clear) and you have turned polarity on the subject thoroughly. Give the instructions to the client to break all contacts, all agreements, all resistance to, all judgments connected, release all projections, and release being the effect of ___(the subject)___ and set a new postulate for how life is NOW.

Living as God/Goddess is a learned activity

Ask the client to set a new postulate to guide the future in the here and now. The aspirant's responsibility is to live in the here and now, living from a new point of view and action.

As we speak, act, and demonstrate

As the aspirant becomes more conscious, as he/she becomes more awake and takes more responsibility for their own words and actions, their speech, actions to self and actions to others, and deeds, he/she will climb to a higher (vibration) level of greatness for themselves and the greatest number of all sentient beings. Look for renewed creativity, with ease and joy. Godhood is at hand.

As explained earlier, it all starts with relaxation, including relaxation techniques of breathing and mindfulness of acceptance and complete allowance. Standing mediation and self-removal of illness, disease, and discomfort will allow one to be totally relaxed, healed, and able to move on. Without relaxation, one may find we use force, concentrated energy, focus, and at the same time decrease our energy and our natural abilities, thereby making the game that much harder to play, and to play and win.

The purpose of this incarnation is *spirituality* and for

one to finally come back to the original realization of who one is; take back your power; live in perfect creativity, peace, joy, Love, and harmony; and allow oneself total happiness in one's creativity. I am God and so are you, and so it is.

Each that have come to the place where one can relate to, but not accept one's Godliness, one must process that immediately. The practitioner's job is to find all distractions that lead one from God/Goddess-hood and allow one the full renewed realization of who one is and not pretending to be.

God/Goddess-hood and so it is…

Thank you for reading *The Gift of Touch.* Now, this is your time in this place for freedom, realization, and the final outcome…

In God Love, Peace, and Joy in Your House

Jay North aka J. Mountain Chief

Please send your friends to his websites: http://www.OneGlobePress.com in Ask them to purchase and download one of Jay's books today.

GLOSSARY

Definitions of Key Words and Phrases

Allowance = Allow to flow, allow to occur, willing to experience.

Aspirant = One who chooses to seek the unfoldment of their soul.

Beingness = The causative creation of <u>Be. The willingness to Be.</u>

Charge = An item that contains negative energy blocks, locks, and barriers. It also refers to the amount of attention given or drawn to an item by the client. People with fixed attention tend to have a lot of "charge" on a subject.

Disconnection = In order for one to be free, one must disconnect from old habits, thoughts and so on, without the need to re-create that which binds or holds one back from the true destiny—unfoldment.

DNA Code = A wrapped, in-capsulated implant that contains a death postulate.

Esoteric level = The deep or high levels of processing that lead one to the final goal. Practiced in many cultures as mysticism.

Form and structure = Solidity = more mass. More mass = less fun.

Four flows = Experienced by self, self to others, others to others, others to self.

GE = Genetic entity. Genes are believed to be responsible for the optimum running of the body. The genetic entity is an implanted reality based on opinion, not on truth or its power.

Implants = Forced-in considerations, conclusions, beliefs, and postulates, either agreed to or resisted upon. They are what entrap a being into not knowing.

IN = Held in, as in trapped.

In-capsulated = The smallest of the cells, a hidden and egg-shaped cell. Its purpose is to make less of.

Karma cleansing = Clearing the energy field of negative past life actions. Principle of cause, effect, and reversal to no effect in the here and now.

Mass = Heavy energy containing weight, form, color, taste, and smell.

Mobius Strip syndrome = A figure eight on its side, running into infinity, never ending, always on the same path.

Money = A tool used for exchange. It is nothing more than energy we use to exchange for more energy

Open memory = Ability to use recall at free will for your entire life tract.

Optimum level = Level which is best, of most value, and of highest productivity and joy.

POCTP = Point of creation, turn polarity. All can be turned if they are undesirable and released. Refer to the separate definitions for "point of creation" and "turn polarity."

Point of creation = All incidents, all that occurs, all items of interest we are looking for have a point of creation, an origin.

Postulate = A decision or conclusion based on past data to help guide one's future or "nowness."

Process = A period of time devoted to handing negative life energies.

Pull = To remove.

Run these commands and phrases and any others you find = Process them to completion so there is no charge remaining.

Solidity = Mass/weight, to be solid.

Solo Processing = Working on one's own body to relieve suffering.

T = Triumph. It means living, doing the heretofore thought impossible.

The Federation = A historical society (organization) of long standing or long time tract; an evil empire. They refer to themselves as royalty. Their mission is power and control. Evidence of their power is experienced through domination, high cost-of-living, a high or outrageous tax system, unjust laws that only protect the wealthy. Prison systems, world banking, global business, oil, and industrialized war machine are their tools used to control others.

Turn polarity = All subjects have polarity (i.e., good and bad, dark and light, etc.). Turning polarity causes the charge from polarity to dissipate completely.

Vibrate it = Create the energy vibration by the way you want it to FEEL

One Globe Press, P.O. BOX 1211, Ojai, California 93024

Jay is available for seminars and phone consultations. Send requests to the address above or E-mail Jay directly at: jaysbookshere@gmail.com

Other Books by Jay North are available at www.oneGlobePress.com ,

Advances Breakthroughs in Massage Technology—N/A

The Windowsill Organic Gardener: Organic Growing for the Urban
    Gardener

Getting Started in Organic Gardening for Fun and Profit

Grow Yourself Rich, a book about marketing organic produce or any
    product, for that matter

Guide to Cooking with Edible Flowers, a self-published guide that
    sold 100,000 copies

The Gift of Touch, a book on massage and energy healing

How to Cure and Prevent Baldness, a Beauty and Barber Industry
    Booklet

Miracles in the Kitchen, comprehensive data on healthy living

Life and Times of a Hollywood Hair Dresser, Confessions of a
    Hollywood Hairdresser—a work in progress

Walter's Big Adventure

Coming soon, six new books:

Open Spaces—The Final Chapter

Living off the Land Organically

How Safe is Your Food?

In Service of Her God: A true story of devoted service, the life of
    Pamela North

Many Roads Traveled, The True Story of North's blood Grandfather
    fleeing oppressive Russia during the revolution of the early 1900's

What Really Happened, the true story of the sixties as Jay North lived
    through them.

Preach Peace—*One Globe Press*

Books by Jay North can also be found on his websites
www.GoingOrganic.com, www.OneGlobePress.com,
www.Amazon.com.

Open Spaces: My Life With Leonard J. Mountain Chief
Leonard's messages are especially important for today's
troubled world $19.95

Miracles In the Kitchen
There is nothing that cannot be cure—naturally, everything
you need for healing in
One complete source $24.95

The Gift Of Touch: Massage Therapy and Energy Healing
Revolutionary new healing techniques $19.95

***The Windowsill Organic Gardener: Organic Gardening
For The Urban Grower***
Yes, absolutely you can grow tomatoes in your kitchen and
just about everything else you enjoy eating $14.95

Grow Yourself Rich: A Marketing Manual
Learn from over forty years experience in marketing $24.95

Guide To Cooking With Edible Flowers N/A

Getting Started in Organic Gardening For Fun And Profit
Now anyone can develop a green thumb with organic
gardening made easy 9.95

Walter's Big Adventure

Walter and Jay take you through life with humor and insight only Westies have $9.95

How To Cure and Prevent Baldness
Want to keep you hair on? This is a must $2.00

How To Grow Cannabis—Organically and Legally
Simple approach to growing simple plants, but guaranteed to be the world's best bud $3.95

How To Cure Cancer Naturally
This is what the AMA does not want you to know $2.00

100 Simple Steps To Perfect Health and Spiritual Fulfillment
A handy booklet for daily healthful living $1.00

In Cases of Severe Health Challenges
Aimed to not only relieve suffering but heal as well $1.00
More to come soon;

What Really Happened—The True Story of The Sixties

Confessions of a Hollywood Hair Dresser

Many Roads Traveled—The Escape of Two Hundred and Fifty Jews from Russia during the Revolution—based on true story of Jay's grandfather

In Service of Her God—True Life Account of Jays Former wife Pamela in Service to Her God

Walter's Big Adventure, II and III

Return to Open Spaces: The final chapter with Jay and

Leonard

Made in the USA
Las Vegas, NV
13 February 2022

43878116R00167